OUTCOMES

SIMULATION
DESIGN
CHARACTERISTICS

SIMULATION IN
NURSING EDUCATION
FROM CONCEPTUALIZATION TO EVALUATION

TEACHER

STUDENT

EDUCATIONAL
PRACTICES

Pamela R. Jeffries, DNS, RN, FAAN
Editor

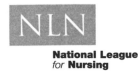

National League for Nursing
61 Broadway
New York, NY 10006
212-363-5555 or 800-669-1656
www.nln.org

ISBN 0-9779557-4-5

Cover design by Brian Vigorita
Art Director, Laerdal Medical Corporation

Figure 3-1 modified and included with permission of
the National League for Nursing, New York, NY

Figures 8-1, 8-2, and 8-3 courtesy of
RCG Architects, Baltimore, MD

Figures 8-1, 8-2, and 8-3 included with permission of
the University of Maryland School of Nursing, Baltimore, MD

This publication has been proudly supported by
Laerdal Medical Corporation

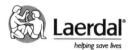

Laerdal®
helping save lives

The authors of this publication exercised full control over the content of each chapter.

Many specific products are mentioned throughout this publication. Such mention does not imply endorsement by the National League for Nursing.

Printed in the United States of America

SIMULATION IN NURSING EDUCATION
FROM CONCEPTUALIZATION TO EVALUATION

TABLE OF CONTENTS

LIST OF FIGURES & TABLES

LIST OF FIGURES

LIST OF TABLES

FOREWORD

The health care system for which nurse educators are preparing students and developing nurses is increasingly complex. Governmental groups and professional organizations call for nurse educators to prepare nurses to be able to access and synthesize knowledge; to integrate evidence into practice; to work collaboratively and in interdisciplinary teams; to use clinical information and decision support systems; and to provide safe and ethical care. Current educational programs and pedagogical approaches are no longer sufficient; clearly, we need new ways of educating our nurses for today's realities.

Simulation is one strategy that holds promise for preparing learners for the complexities of clinical practice. Well-designed simulations set the stage for students to work with authentic problems, synthesize data, make clinical decisions, and reflect on their practice. Because simulations take place in the safety of the simulation center, risk to clients is eliminated and learning becomes paramount. Simulations have the power to reshape teaching and learning as nurse educators serve as the designers of the learning activity, rather than the dispensers of facts; become coaches instead of lecturers; and hone their teaching skills to guide learners to reflect and critically evaluate their care. At the same time, students become active learners, abandoning memorization for accessing knowledge, and thinking and applying learning in context rather than provide answers to fact-based tests.

Simulation in Nursing Education comes to us at an opportune time as nurse educators are redesigning educational programs and reconsidering the most effective ways to teach today's students. The authors of this book provide an evidence-based, framework-driven approach to designing, implementing, and evaluating the use of simulations in nursing education. The book guides the reader through the simulation design process, offers suggestions for setting up the simulation center, tells us how to integrate best practices in teaching and learning, and provides tools to evaluate the effectiveness of the simulation. In short, this book is a personal faculty development plan! Finally, the authors encourage us to engage in the scholarship of teaching and learning and provide direction for further testing the impact of simulation as a strategy for preparing nurses for clinical practice in a variety of settings.

Simulation in Nursing Education is written by our colleagues, who, for the last three years, have been immersed in developing and testing a framework for creating and using simulations. It is rare to have a book that offers field-tested strategies. The authors have given us a gift — it is ours to open and use.

Diane M. Billings, EdD, RN, FAAN
Chancellor's Professor Emeritus
Indiana University School of Nursing
Indianapolis, Indiana

PREFACE

In 2003, the National League for Nursing and the Laerdal Corporation entered into an alliance to conduct a national, multisite, multimethod study of the use of simulation in nursing education. The specific purposes of this study were to (a) develop and test models that nursing faculty can implement when using simulation to promote student learning, (b) develop a cadre of nursing faculty who can use simulation in innovative ways to enhance student learning, (c) contribute to the refinement of the body of knowledge about the use of simulation in nursing education, and (d) demonstrate the value of collaboration between the corporate and not-for-profit worlds.

The project was led by a team of individuals including a project director, a project coordinator at each of eight schools selected to participate, NLN's senior director for professional development, and Laerdal's regional director, west/central. Over the course of three years, the team developed a framework to guide their work, developed and pilot tested two research instruments, collected and analyzed data from each site, and reported their findings to various groups of educators. The final report on this project is included in this book as Appendix A.

The chapters in this book were written by the members of the project team and, in some instances, colleagues at project coordinators' schools. They make frequent reference to the NLN/Laerdal Simulation Study, so reviewing the final report may be helpful prior to reading the text.

Nurse educators are facing great challenges today in keeping up with the demands required to prepare nursing graduates for 21st century health care practice. Health care environments are complex, and they require high-tech, problem-solving, and decision-making skills, as well as a strong knowledge background. Faculty must consider all these factors when preparing students for clinical practice. The shortage of nurse educators, the explosion of advanced technologies in education, and diminished financial resources are additional challenges facing nursing education. Confronting these changes and challenges, nurse educators are exploring new teaching-learning methods, clinical models, and educational practices to provide high quality education to nursing students.

As they explore innovative models and ways to increase students' clinical diagnostic skills, nursing faculty are increasingly designing, using, and implementing simulations as an essential part of the educational experience. Clinical simulations are activities or events that replicate real-life experiences, and they are currently being used to enhance or supplement learning in classroom, laboratory, and clinical settings. Simulations also are being used for student remediation on selected skills, to assess students' clinical competencies and decision-making skills, and to orient students to clinical challenges such as bioterrorism that they may not encounter directly but for which they need to be prepared.

The use of simulations requires faculty in all types of programs to reexamine their teaching-learning practices, curriculum designs, and evaluation strategies, as traditional ways of designing and delivering nursing education may no longer be relevant with the incorporation of this advanced technology for teaching and learning. When incorporating simulations into nursing education, faculty need to consider the following:

- Being prepared with skills and knowledge to design a high quality simulation

- Understanding how to implement a clinical simulation so students can achieve the learning outcomes desired

- Participating in the shift from a teacher-centered to a student-centered focus that is interactive and experiential

- Assuring there is faculty development for educators learning to use simulations in the teaching-learning environment

- Promoting the initiation of collaborative partnerships and consortiums so educators can "work smarter" and more efficiently by, for example, sharing case scenarios, programming, and design elements

- Developing an evaluation plan to measure learning outcomes, ensuring that simulations are achieving the competencies desired

- Initiating a research plan so this educational technology can be studied in a way that will contribute to the science of nursing education

We have written this book on simulation for nurse educators preparing to use or wishing to expand and enhance the use of simulation in the teaching-learning process. The book is also for educators in the service sector who are looking for methods to assess the competency of new graduates, to recertify employees in certain skill sets, or to teach about a product or skill associated with a new policy or practice before implementing it in the actual health care environment.

With each chapter providing foundational content that can help educators get started with clinical simulations, we intend this to be a guide and resource for developing, implementing, and evaluating those simulations. Our hope is that this book will inspire and engage educators to use simulation in nursing education and give them the foundation that can be built upon to enhance professional growth in this area of education.

Nursing education is in a time of dramatic change and challenge — a time that is exciting and filled with many opportunities to influence the discipline of nursing. We believe that the material here will encourage educators to get started with simulations or to take the next step in using simulations in nursing education that will lead to a new model for high-quality teaching-learning and clinical education.

Pamela R. Jeffries
Indianapolis, Indiana
November 20, 2006

ACKNOWLEDGMENTS

Many individuals have been involved in making this publication a reality. First, sincere thanks go to the contributing authors, most of whom were the Project Coordinators during the three-year, multisite National League for Nursing (NLN)/Laerdal Simulation Study and who shared their knowledge and expertise, as well as their passion and motivation, about simulations and nursing education. These individuals, who truly are simulation specialists and mentors, include the following: Janis C. Childs, Reba Moyer Childress, Cheryl Feken Dixon, Mitzi Horn, Marcy Hovancsek, Ruth Politi, Kristen Rogers, and Debra Spunt. Additional thanks are extended to Nina Carter, Susan B. Sepples, and Kristy Chambers.

We also want to thank Mary Anne Rizzolo, senior director for professional development at the National League for Nursing, who has been the facilitator, liaison, coach, and "guide on the side" throughout the three-year project. She helped keep the project on task and helped me and the project coordinators achieve the goals we set at the start of and throughout our three years together. In addition, many thanks to Terry Valiga, chief program officer at the National League for Nursing, who played a major role in helping us assemble and publish this book. Without her assistance, the book would not have been possible.

Many thanks as well to three key Laerdal colleagues: Tore Laerdal, CEO; Rosie Patterson, regional director, west/central; and Marion Young, manager for public relations and media. Each of these individuals provided support and assistance, conveyed confidence in the project team, and believed in the endeavor. We greatly appreciated their willingness to allow this project to become a reality. In addition, we would like to thank Jay Ober, Director of the International Academy for Clinical Simulation and Research at the University of Miami, for the expertise and wisdom he provided on the simulation project.

We thank our families and colleagues for their continued love, support, patience, and encouragement throughout this undertaking. A special thanks, too, to my dean and the deans of the eight schools of nursing involved in the project for their support and encouragement throughout the three-year simulation study. Finally, we wish to thank the many students and faculty who participated in the research and continue to be our major focus in nursing education.

P.R.J.

DEDICATION

This book is dedicated to our colleagues in education whom we hope to empower to design and implement simulations in the teaching-learning environment. It also is dedicated to our students who stimulate us to explore new teaching-learning strategies to keep them engaged, provide realistic experiences, and improve learning outcomes.

CHAPTER 1

USING SIMULATIONS IN NURSING EDUCATION

Marcella T. Hovancsek, MSN, RN

"I hear and I forget. I see and I remember.

I do and I understand."

Confucius

More than 2,500 years ago, Confucius offered wisdom on the educational merits of performance practice and experiential learning, and we continue to benefit from those insights today. Indeed, high fidelity simulation technology has proliferated over the last decade, and the use of simulation in health care and in daily life is extensive. For example, in an effort to educate students who will go to their senior prom, fire and police departments, with the assistance of medical flight professionals, enact simulated alcohol-related motor vehicle accidents using high-school students as the "victims." Hurricane Katrina motivated officials in many at-risk cities to practice partial and total evacuation using computer-based exercises. In addition, health care educators are investing in technology to ensure that their learning and simulation centers are venues where students can participate in clinically accurate and risk-free simulations that will best prepare them for the realities of the environments in which they will practice. But what is simulation, and why is it important in the education of nurses?

USE OF SIMULATION IN HEALTH CARE EDUCATION

The first simulation models used in health care education came on the scene in the 1960s with the introduction of "Resusci® Anne" (a resuscitation trainer) and "Harvey" (a full-sized mannequin designed to train professionals in cardiology) (Cooper & Taqueti, 2004). Cooper and Taqueti also found, in a study done in the 1980s of 208 medical students who were either trained at the bedside or trained with "Harvey," that those trained on the "Harvey" simulator showed enhanced skill at correctly performing cardiac assessments at the bedside and an enhanced sense of confidence in their ability.

During the 1980s, anesthesia educators studied how simulation was being used in aviation training and in military training directed at team and individual performance during critical events, and they created a simulated training environment for anesthesia administration. The final decade of the 20th century was a landmark one for simulation development for health care with the birth of the World Wide Web and the Virtual Human Project (Rosen, 2004). Without a doubt, the introduction of affordable, portable, and versatile human patient simulators in the late 1990s transformed health care education and is the technology of the future for competency testing and continuing education.

EVOLUTION OF NURSING AS A PRACTICED-BASED DISCIPLINE

During Nightingale's time and up to the middle of the twentieth century, the most valued attributes of nurses were efficiency, keen observational skills, tenderness, an effort to ensure comfort, and attention to the hygiene needs of patients (Bjork, 1999). During World War II, nurses were called upon to take on more sophisticated clinical skills, such as the initiation and monitoring of intravenous infusions (Campbell & Lunn, 1997), and the nursing role began to evolve in its complexity. At the same time, the education of nurses shifted from a hospital-based apprenticeship model to collegiate programs, and we witnessed the proliferation of community colleges since the 1950s and the growth of baccalaureate programs. Skills laboratories were created in many of these programs to help students apply the theory learned in the classroom in a relatively safe environment prior to facing the challenges presented by the clinical setting.

In addition to these changes, the era following the end of World War II was filled with tremendous advances in patient care technology. The science of resuscitation was developed, the external defibrillator was invented, pacemaker technology was introduced, and the ability to provide positive pressure ventilation was established (Rosen). Providing patient care held new challenges for nurses, and they needed to be prepared to face such challenges. Simulation was part of the answer.

DEFINING SIMULATION

A simulation resembles reality. In specific reference to health care, simulation is an attempt "to replicate some or nearly all of the essential aspects of a clinical situation so that the situation may be more readily understood and managed when it occurs for real in clinical practice" (Morton, 1995, p. 76). Simulations are described along a continuum — from low-fidelity to high-fidelity — regarding the degree to which they approach reality. On the low-fidelity end of the simulation spectrum are experiences such as using case studies to educate students about patient situations or using role-play to immerse students in a particular clinical situation. Farther along the continuum are partial task trainers, such as IV cannulation arms or low-technology mannequins, that are used to help students practice specific psychomotor skills that are integral to patient care. More technologically sophisticated are computer-based simulations in which the participant relies on a two-dimensional focused experience to problem solve, perform a skill, and/or make decisions during the clinical scenario. Finally, full-scale, high-fidelity patient simulators are extremely realistic and sophisticated and provide a high level of interactivity and realism for the learner.

Health care educators have learned from the experiences of colleagues in the military and aviation who have trained individuals in this manner since the 1970s. Like military strategizing and flying a plane, making sound decisions in unpredictable health care situations requires critical thinking, time-sensitive action, and skilled task performance (Macedonia, Gherman, & Satin, 2003). Simulation offers health care educators a tool that can be used repeatedly by learners who need sequential experiences or less frequently for those who are more experienced. It also serves as a medium to provide a wide range of experiences that are either too rare or too risky for novices to engage in using actual patients.

PREPARATION OF BEGINNING STUDENTS
FOR CLINICAL PRACTICE

Today, simulation is not reserved for highly experienced individuals (e.g., pilots, military strategists, anesthesiologists). It also is being used to support the learning of beginning students. In nursing, where high patient acuity levels, shortened patient stays, and critical staffing shortages make the clinical environment an incredibly stressful one for the beginning student, low-fidelity simulated experiences are being used. With these task trainers or standard mannequins, beginning students are able to practice skills and care giving in a safe environment that allows them to make mistakes, learn from those mistakes, and develop confidence in their ability to approach patients and practice in the clinical setting.

As they progress through their programs, nursing students participate in high-fidelity simulation experiences that help them develop and practice decision making skills that previously were acquired only as a result of the careful attention of a clinical instructor or staff preceptor, or by luck (Rauen, 2001). Human simulators, for example, are able to provide a wide range of complex cardiac rhythms, variations in QRS morphology, changes in blood pressure, normal and abnormal breath sounds and patterns, pulses, and bowel sounds. They also can provide computer-generated subjective information such as audible groans. By using a programmed scenario that simulates respiratory arrest or aberrant cardiac rhythm, for example, students can demonstrate their ability to establish priorities, make decisions, take appropriate action, and work successfully as part of a team. While using simulation, students are able to learn from and correct their mistakes without the mistakes adversely affecting live patients and without teachers or clinical instructors needing to step in, correct, and control the situation. Students can repeatedly practice a scenario and use the simulation for remediation purposes, both of which enhance students' preparation for clinical practice.

USING SIMULATION AS AN ASSESSMENT
OR EVALUATION METHOD

At this time, simulation is used far more frequently as a teaching strategy than as an evaluation or assessment method in nursing. The literature does reveal, however, that simulation is being used in the performance assessment of anesthesiologists (Schuwirth & van der Vleuten, 2003), as well as for the evaluation and remediation, if necessary, of those physicians who have been identified as incompetent. For example, the New York State Society of Anesthesiologists, in response to an already established state physician-monitoring program, now uses human patient simulators to evaluate and remediate anesthesiologists with lapsed skills (Rosenblatt, Abrams, & the New York State Society of Anesthesiologists, 2002).

Despite the fact that simulated methods of assessment or evaluation of competence have not been rigorously tested for validity or reliability, it is expected that simulation will be used in the future to provide useful information regarding the clinical reasoning, record keeping, and technical skills of individuals. In nursing, we are likely to see an increase in the use of simulation to measure progress toward programmatic goals (i.e., low-stakes assessment) and to measure competence for licensure, certification, or performance appraisals (i.e., high-stakes assessment) (Jeffries, Hovancsek, & Clochesy, 2005). Indeed, the use of clinical simulation testing has been considered by the National Council of State Boards of Nursing as a possible future component of the National Council Licensure Examination for Registered Nurses (NCLEX-RN®) (Johnson, Zerwic, & Theis, 1999).

Advantages to Using Simulation

It is not enough for nurse educators to include simulation in their courses because it is popular, available, or "trendy." Instead it is important to use simulation for its advantages related to student learning. A simulation experience allows students to critically analyze their own actions (or failure to act), reflect on their own skill sets, and critique the clinical decisions of others (Jeffries et al.; Rauen). Students may repeat the experience to enhance learning, based on an analysis of their mistakes, the feedback provided by the instructor, or the immediate feedback function of some sophisticated computer-assisted simulation equipment.

Another advantage to using simulation is that the instructor does not take over, as often happens on an actual clinical unit when students are mishandling a situation or having difficulty with a skill. In simulated situations, students are allowed to make mistakes and then are guided to turn them into opportunities from which skills, knowledge and, in some cases, ability to work as a team member grow (Johnson et al.). Research has shown that students involved in active learning retain knowledge longer (Johnson et al.), and simulated learning is active learning. In addition, simulation allows instructors to expose students to clinical experiences they would rarely see (e.g., acute severe asthma or cerebral vascular accident). Finally, students, once they are accustomed to simulation experiences, report a decreased level of performance anxiety and a heightened sense of self-confidence in their psychomotor skills and critical thinking abilities (Jamison, Hovancsek, & Clochesy, 2006; Jeffries, 2005).

Challenges of Using Simulation

The challenges of using simulation in nursing education appear to present themselves to administrators of schools of nursing and faculty more than to students. Practical challenges of using simulation include expense, space, computer literacy, and technical support (Rauen). Faculty time issues and the need for more research to validate simulation as a teaching-learning strategy or assessment/evaluation method that makes a difference in student learning and positive patient outcomes complete the list.

The development of simulation-enhanced education is costly and includes the fixed cost of the equipment (patient simulator or partial task trainers) and the costs associated with operating, maintaining, troubleshooting, and repairing it (Morgan & DeSousa, 2004). In addition, since simulation is integrated into more and more courses or used routinely for assessment and evaluation, there is likely to be a need for a simulation center coordinator and technical support personnel (Morgan & De Sousa; Rauen).

When a computer-assisted patient simulator is purchased, space often becomes an issue. Not only is adequate space needed for the life-sized simulator itself, but additional space is required for the supporting equipment (e.g., the ventilator) needed during the simulated situation. Further spatial challenges include an area needed for the participants and observers, a remote area for the debriefing (reflective thinking) session, storage space for supporting props and equipment, and a control area from where the simulation may be staged (Olympio, 2004).

For more than two decades, nurse educators have realized that computer literacy and accompanying technical computer proficiency are essential for faculty and students (Newbern, 1985; Richard, 1997). With the proliferating use of simulation, particularly high-fidelity simulation, nurse educators now find that the faculty must at least understand the basics of operating and programming this highly complex, sophisticated piece of equipment.

Time requirements provide additional challenges to educators using simulation. Developing simulation scenarios is time-intensive, comparable to the time needed to develop a complex lecture (Rauen). However, because the use of simulation involves a paradigm shift from a teacher-centered to a learner-centered experience, the creation of the scenario itself is only the first step. Educators also must envision and plan for the varied learner responses that may occur during the experience (Jeffries et al.). In addition, since only a small number of learners (participants and observers) can take part in a simulated experience at one time, faculty must plan to offer the simulation repeatedly (Rauen).

An overarching challenge to the future of simulation in nursing and health care education is to validate whether it makes a difference when compared to more traditional approaches to helping students learn safe and competent care of patients (Greenberg, 2004). Because simulation is in its nascent stage, future research is needed to establish this form of education as financially and educationally sound.

SUMMARY AND CONCLUSION

The range of simulation technology that is available to nurse educators continues to expand, and ways in which this technology is being used as a tool to prepare nurses for competent practice that meets the health care needs of patients are evolving. Since nursing is a practiced-based discipline and the technological advances that have occurred in patient care and in simulation over the last half century are exploding, nurse educators must be aware of the advantages and the challenges of using simulation as a teaching/learning/evaluation strategy and use this tool effectively.

Simulation holds promise as an essential strategy in the education of nurses, and more research is needed to validate its worth as a teaching and assessment/evaluation method. The chapters that follow are designed to help nurse educators design, implement, and evaluate simulations, form alliances to support simulated learning in nursing, and ask significant questions for future study.

REFERENCES

Bjork, I. T. (1999). What constitutes a nursing practical skill? Western Journal of Nursing Research, 21(1), 51-69.

Campbell, T., & Lunn, D. (1997). Intravenous therapy: Current practice and nursing concerns. British Journal of Nursing, 6(21), 1218-1228.

Cooper, J.B., & Taqueti, V.R. (2004). A brief history of the development of mannequin simulators for clinical education and training. Quality & Safety in Health Care, 13 (suppl1), i11-i18.

Greenberg, R. (2004). Technology-enhanced simulation: Looking ahead to 2020. In G. E. Loyd, C. L. Lake, & R. B. Greenberg, Practical health care simulations (pp. 575-580). Philadelphia: Elsevier.

Jamison, R. J., Hovancsek, M. T., & Clochesy, J. M. (2006), A pilot study assessing simulation using two simulation methods for teaching intravenous cannulation. Clinical Simulation in Nursing Education, 2(1). Available from the International Nursing Association for Clinical Simulation and Learning, www.inacsl.org.

Jeffries, P. R. (2005). A framework for designing, implementing, and evaluating simulations used as teaching strategies in nursing. Nursing Education Perspectives, 26(2), 96-103.

Jeffries P. R., Hovancsek M. T., & Clochesy J. M. (2005). Using clinical simulations in distance education. In J. M. Novotny, & R. H. Davis (Eds.), Distance education in nursing (2nd ed.) (pp. 83-99). New York: Springer Publishing.

Johnson, J. H., Zerwic, J. J., & Theis, S. L. (1999). Clinical simulation laboratory: An adjunct to clinical teaching. Nurse Educator, 24(5), 37-41.

Macedonia, C. R. Gherman, R. B., & Satin, A. J. (2003). Simulation laboratories for training in obstetrics and gynecology. The American College of Obstetrics and Gynecology, 102(2), 388-391.

Morgan, P. J., & DeSousa, S. L. (2004). Human considerations in healthcare simulation. In G. E. Loyd, C. L. Lake, & R. B. Greenberg, Practical health care simulations (pp.75-85). Philadelphia: Elsevier.

Morton, P. G. (1995). Creating a laboratory that simulates the critical care environment. Critical Care Nurse, 16(6), 76-81.

Newbern, V. B. (1985). Computer literacy in nursing education. An overview. *Nursing Clinics of North America, 20*(3), 549-556.

Olympio, M. A. (2004). Space considerations in healthcare simulation. In G. E. Loyd, C. L. Lake, & R. B. Greenberg, *Practical health care simulations* (pp. 49-74). Philadelphia: Elsevier.

Rauen, C. A. (2001). Using simulation to teach critical thinking skills. *Critical Care Nursing Clinics of North America, 13*(1), 93-103.

Richard, P. L. (1997). Conquering technophobia: Preparing faculty for today. *Student Health Technology Information, 46*, 437-441.

Rosen, K. R. (2004). The history of medical simulation. In G. E. Loyd, C. L. Lake, & R. B. Greenberg, *Practical health care simulations* (pp. 3-21). Philadelphia: Elsevier.

Rosenblatt, M. A., Abrams, K. J., & the New York State Society of Anesthesiologists. (2002). The use of the human patient simulator in the evaluation of and development of a remedial prescription for an anesthesiologist with lapsed medical skills. *Anesthesia Analgesia, 94*, 149-153.

Schuwirth, L. W., & van der Vleuten, C. P. (2003). The use of clinical simulations in assessment. *Medical Education, 37*(suppl 1), S65-S71.

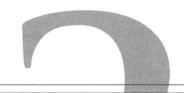

CHAPTER 2
SIMULATIONS: EDUCATION AND ETHICS
Sharon Decker, MSN, RN, CCRN, CS

"To know how to suggest is the great art of teaching."

Henri Frederic Amiel

Patient safety is a major societal issue and is receiving attention from federal commissions, accreditation organizations, health care agencies, and consumer advocacy groups. The importance of the patient safety issue in the health care industry is validated by multiple studies, and major causes of safety concerns have been identified. The cause of inadvertent harm to patients has been associated with ineffective communication between health care providers and inadequate orientation (Leonard, Graham, & Bonacum, 2004). For example, inadequate orientation of health care providers was identified as the underlying cause of 87% of deaths related to mechanical ventilation, and communication breakdown between health care providers accounts for 76% of deaths in such situations (JCAHO, 2002).

Kohn, Corrigan, and Donaldson (1999) stress "...it is simply not acceptable for patients to be harmed by the same health care system that is supposed to offer healing and comfort" (p. 3). The reality, however, is that the demand on health care providers has become more complex with the advancement of technology (Koerner, 2003; Long, 2004), the increasing complexity of patient care situations, the need for rapid decision making despite conflicting or incomplete information, and increasing interdependence among members of the health care team (Hamman, 2004; Maddox, Wakefield, & Bull, 2001). Such realities challenge educators in the health professions to design teaching, learning, and evaluation strategies that enhance students' abilities to practice safely and effectively in this health care environment. Among the strategies suggested to assist educators in meeting student learning needs and developing their practice competencies are e-learning, virtual reality, and scenario-based simulation (Koerner; Ziv, Wolpe, Small, & Glick, 2003). The use of scenario-based simulation holds exceptional promise for education, particularly for the education of nurses.

The use of simulation as a tool to assist in resolving the patient safety issue while promoting students' learning is identified in the Commonwealth Fund report (2003). This national report recommends "the use of simulation at all levels of the education experience, from students' first encounters with clinical care to continuing education and certification of master clinicians" (p. 44). The National Council of State Boards of Nursing (NCSBN) (2005) predicts the future of clinical education in nursing will include increased use of simulation. Simulation as defined by the NCSBN is an educational process that imitates the working environment and requires the learner to demonstrate procedural techniques, decision making, and critical thinking. In addition, the NCSBN challenges nurse faculty to "focus on the quality" of actual patient experiences "not the numbers" (p. 8).

ETHICAL CONSIDERATIONS

The identified societal issues of patient safety and the challenge to promote student learning and competency through increased use of simulation require nurse educators to consider the ethical considerations of integrating simulation as an educational strategy in the teaching, learning, and evaluation process. Possible questions to consider are presented in Table 2-1.

Table 2-1. Thoughtful Questions to Consider
1. Would the inequity in social justice be minimized if health care students were prepared and competencies validated through simulation prior to providing patient care?
2. Would the inequity in social justice be decreased if simulation were used to promote and validate interdisciplinary teamwork?
3. Would the principle of autonomy be violated when informed consents do not provide full disclosure of all pertinent information?
4. When informed consent is attained for a procedure, should a patient be provided with the qualifications of the student performing the procedure?
5. What is the responsibility of faculty related to the use of simulation in the educational process, in light of research that validates that simulation promotes student learning while promoting a humanistic outlook toward patients?
6. Would learning through simulation prior to patient contact promote the competence of health care providers and thereby decrease the overuse of services?
7. Does simulation provide a valid and reliable method to evaluate a student's competence and, if so, what is the educator's obligation related to incorporating this technique into the evaluation process?
8. Is the act of not integrating simulation into the educational process of the health care student a form of neglect and, if so, could this cause an ethos of distrust (with both students and patients) and compromise the purpose of professional relationships?
9. Are nurse educators and other health care professionals demonstrating compassion when they allow students to perform procedures for the first time on clients instead of first providing students with simulated experiences?
10. In the future, will students be required to demonstrate specific competencies prior to engaging in actual patient care?

THE PRINCIPLE OF JUSTICE

Justice as defined by Beauchamp and Childress (2001) is fairness or the "appropriate treatment in light of what is due or owed to persons" (p. 226). Social justice according to Beauchamp and Childress requires individuals to share equally in the benefits and risks of medical innovations, research, and practitioner training. Ziv and colleagues (2003) acknowledge that some citizens may be bearing a disproportionate amount of the benefits and risks related to practitioner training. Therefore, since research has demonstrated students perceive an increase in critical thinking skills (Henrichs, Rule, Grady, & Ellis, 2002; Rhodes & Curran, 2005) and the retention of knowledge specifically related to performing procedures (Henrichs et al.; Issenberg, McGaghie, Hart, Mayer, Felner, & Petrusa, 1999), should educators ask, "Would the inequity in social justice be minimized if health care students are prepared and competencies validated through simulation prior to providing patient care?"

Kohn and colleagues identify the need to enhance teamwork within the health professions in an effort to promote mutual commitment and patient safety. For example, a study conducted by one team (Shapiro, Morey, Small, Langford, Kayor, Jagminas, Suner, Salisbury, Simon, & Jay, 2004) demonstrates an improvement in clinical team performance when simulation using a patient simulator was integrated into an existing didactic teamwork curriculum. Therefore, another question to be considered is, "Would the inequity in social justice be decreased if simulation were used to promote and validate interdisciplinary teamwork?"

THE PRINCIPLE OF AUTONOMY

Autonomy includes respect and acknowledges an individual's decision-making rights. Beauchamp and Childress state "respect for autonomy is not a mere ideal in health care; it is a professional obligation" (p. 63). Autonomous choice, according to Beauchamp and Childress, "is a right, not a duty of patients" (p. 63). A question to discuss is, "Would the principle of autonomy be violated when informed consents do not provide full disclosure of all pertinent information?" Beauchamp and Childress also stress that "One gives an informed consent to an intervention if (and perhaps only if) one is competent to act, receives a thorough disclosure, comprehends the disclosure, acts voluntarily, and consents to the interventions" (p. 79). Therefore, should educators ask, "When informed consent is obtained for a procedure, should a patient be provided with the qualifications of the student performing the procedure?" For example, should patients be told if a student is performing a venipuncture for the first time?

One could argue that patients admitted to teaching hospitals are generally aware that residents, interns, and nursing and allied health students will be providing direct care. Yet a study by Cohen , McCullough, Kessel, Apostolides, Alden, & Heiderich (1987) revealed that only 37.5 percent of teaching hospitals that responded to the research survey specifically informed patients that students would be participating in their care. In addition, when many of these patients were questioned, they could not distinguish between a student and a health care professional.

The principle of autonomy related to students needs to be addressed when considering the use of simulation as a learning, teaching, and evaluation strategy. Ziv et al. (2003) emphasize that when student autonomy is respected, it leads to better educated students who develop a more humanistic outlook toward patients. Simulation can be used to identify (Morgan, Cleave-Hogg, DeSousa, & Tarshis, 2003; Rhodes & Curran) and support the learning needs of the student (Ziv et al., 2003) and to promote the student's feelings of self-confidence (Bearnson & Wiker, 2005; Henrichs et al.; Jeffries & Rizzolo, 2005). Research validates that simulation promotes student learning while promoting a humanistic outlook toward patients. Should nurse educators be questioning the responsibility of faculty related to the use of simulation in the educational process?

THE PRINCIPLE OF BENEFICENCE

As defined by Beauchamp and Childress, beneficence "refers to an action done to benefit others; benevolence refers to the character trait or virtues of being disposed to act for the benefit of others (the capacity for promoting and achieving good); and principle of beneficence refers to a moral obligation to act for the benefit of others" (p. 166). Beneficence suggests that unwarranted care and the overuse of services should be prevented during patient care. Therefore, a question to be considered is, "Would learning through simulation prior to patient contact promote the competency of the health care providers and thereby decrease the overuse of services?"

THE PRINCIPLE OF NONMALEFICENCE

According to the principle of nonmaleficence an individual ought not to inflict harm that includes emotional, physical, and financial injury (Beauchamp & Childress). Yet, according to Smith and Crawford (2003), many avoidable errors in health care continue to be correlated to inaccessible data and the inability of newly licensed RNs to make clinical decisions based on data obtained from physical assessments and diagnostic tests. Furthermore, *The Code of Ethics for Nurses* (ANA, 2001) stresses, "Nurse educators have a responsibility to ensure that basic competencies are achieved...prior to entry of an individual into practice" (p. 13). Therefore, a question that could be debated is, "Does simulation provide a valid and reliable method to evaluate a student's competency and, if so, what is the educator's obligation related to incorporating this technique into the evaluation process?" For example, Ziv, Small, and Wolpe (2000) stress that the use of patient simulators can provide consistent learning and evaluation of experience, including atypical patterns, rare diseases, critical incidents, near misses, and crises. These experts stress that educators have "an ethical obligation to make all efforts to expose a health professional to clinical challenges that can be reasonably well simulated prior to allowing them to encounter and be responsible for similar real-life challenges" (p. 492).

THE PRINCIPLE OF VERACITY

Veracity is defined by Beauchamp and Childress as not intentionally deceiving or misleading a patient. Pellegrino and Thomasma (1993) stress "trust and self-effacement can be, and must be, indispensable traits of the authentic professional" (p.158). The virtue of trust is acknowledged as central and indispensable to the nurse-patient (or faculty-student) relationship. Peter and Morgan (2001) stress that trust is an obligation, not a privilege, and that without trust, the healing or helping goal cannot be attained. Therefore, a question to be addressed could be, "Is the act of not integrating simulation into the education of the health care students a form of neglect, and if so, could this cause an ethos of distrust (with both students and patients) and compromise the purpose of professional relationships?"

THE PRINCIPLE OF COMPASSION

Compassion is discussed by Pellegrino and Thomasma as an essential virtue in health care delivery. The authors stress that "compassion and competence go hand in hand as necessary and mutually reinforcing virtues"; this is further emphasized by the statement, "nothing is more inconsistent with compassion than the well-meaning, empathetic, but incompetent clinician" (p. 83). Therefore, a question that could be considered is, "Are nurse educators and other healthcare professionals demonstrating compassion when they allow students to perform procedures for the first time on clients instead of first providing students with simulated experiences?"

SUMMARY

As technology advances, computerized simulations will become more realistic and provide students and health care professionals opportunities to learn and remain proficient in most procedures without endangering patient safety. A final question that needs to be addressed is, "In the future, will students be required to demonstrate specific competencies prior to engaging in actual patient care?" Educators are required to ensure patient safety while providing educational opportunities for students to develop the competency needed to provide patient care. Therefore, educators have the responsibility to advocate in the interest of both the student and the patient while promoting change in the culture of nursing education.

REFERENCES

ANA (American Nurses Association). (2001). _Code of ethics for nurses with interpretive standards._ Washington, DC: American Nurses Publishing.

Bearnson, C. S., & Wiker, K. M. (2005). Human patient simulators: A new face in baccalaureate nursing education at Brigham Young University. _Journal of Nursing Education, 44_(9), 421-425.

Beauchamp, T. L., & Childress, J. F. (2001). _Principles of biomedical ethics_ (3rd ed.). Washington DC: Oxford University Press.

Cohen D. L., McCullough, L. B., Kessel, R. W., Apostolides, A. Y., Alden, E. R., & Heiderich, K. L. (1987). Informed consent policies governing medical students' interaction with patients. _Journal of Medical Education, 62_(10), 789-798.

Commonwealth Fund (2003). _Envisioning the future of academic health centers_ (Final report of the Task Force on Academic Health Centers). Washington, DC: National Academy of Science.

Hamman, W. R. (2004, October). The complexity of team training: What we have learned from aviation and its applications to medicine. [Electronic version.] _Quality & Safety in Health Care, 13_(suppl 1), i72-i79. Available: http://qshc.bmj.com/cgi/reprint/13/suppl_1/i72

Henrichs, B., Rule, A., Grady, M., & Ellis, W. (2002). Nurse anesthesia students' perceptions of the anesthesia patient simulator: A qualitative study. _American Association of Nurse Anesthetists Journal, 70_(3), 219-225.

Issenberg, S. B., McGaghie, W. C., Hart, A. R., Mayer, J. W., Felner, J. M., & Petrusa, E. R. (1999). Simulation technology for health care professional skills training and assessment. _Journal of the American Medical Association, 282_(9), 861-866.

JCAHO (Joint Commission on Accreditation of Healthcare Organizations). (2002, February 26). Sentinel Event Alert. Issue 25. [Electronic version.] Available: http://www.jointcommission.org/SentinelEvents/SentinelEventAlert/sea_25.htm.

Jeffries, P., & Rizzolo, M. A. (2005, June). NLN/Laerdal simulation study: Phase III, part 2. Presented at the Study Project Coordinators Meeting, San Antonio, TX.

Koerner, J. G. (2003). The virtues of the virtual world: Enhancing the technology/knowledge professional interface for life-long learning. _Nursing Administration Quarterly, 27_(1), 9-17.

Kohn L., Corrigan, J., & Donaldson, M. (Eds.). (1999). _To err is human: Building a safer health system_. Washington, DC: National Academy of Science.

Leonard, M., Graham, S., & Bonacum, D. (2004). The human factor: The critical importance of effective teamwork and communication in providing safe care. [Electronic version.] _Quality & Safety in Health Care, 13_(suppl 1), i85-i90.
Available: http://qshc.bmj.com/cgi/content/full/13/suppl_1/i85

Long, K. A. (2004). Preparing nurses for the 21st century: Reenvisioning nursing education and practice. _Journal of Professional Nursing, 20_(2), 82-88.

Maddox, P. J., Wakefield, M., & Bull, J. (2001). Patient safety and the need for professional and educational change. _Nursing Outlook, 49_(1), 8-13.

Morgan, P. J., Cleave-Hogg, D., DeSousa, S., & Tarshis, J. (2003). Identification of gaps in the achievement of undergraduate anesthesia educational objectives using high-fidelity patient simulation. _Anesthesia & Analgesia, 97_, 1690-1694.

National Council of State Boards of Nursing. (2005). Clinical instruction in prelicensure nursing programs. [Electronic version.]
Available: https://www.ncsbn.org/Final_Clinical_Instr_Pre_Nsg_programs.pdf

Pellegrino, E. D., & Thomasma, D. C. (1993). _The virtues in medical practice_. New York: Oxford University Press.

Peter, E., & Morgan, K. P. (2001). Exploration of a trust approach for nursing ethics. _Nursing Inquiry, 8_(1), 3-10.

Rhodes, M. L., & Curran, C. (2005). Use of the human patient simulator to teach clinical judgment skills in baccalaureate nursing programs. _Computers in Nursing, 23_(5), 256-262.

Shapiro, M. J., Morey, J. C., Small, S. D., Langford, V., Kayor, C. J., Jagminas, L., Suner, S., Salisbury, M. L. Simon, R., & Jay, G. D. (2004). Simulation based teamwork training for emergency department staff: Does it improve clinical team performance when added to an existing didactic teamwork curriculum? [Electronic version.] _Quality & Safety in Health Care, 13_(6), 417-421. Available: http://qshc.bmj.com/cgi/content/full/13/6/417

Smith, J., & Crawford, L. (2003). *Report of findings from the practice and professional issues survey. National Council of State Boards of Nursing (NCSBN) Research Brief, 7.*

Ziv, A., Small, S. D., & Wolpe, P. R. (2000). *Patient safety and simulation-based medical education. Medical Teacher, 22(5), 489-495.*

Ziv, A., Wolpe, P. R., Small, S. D., & Glick, S. (2003). *Simulation-based medical education: An ethical imperative. Academic Medicine, 78(8), 783-788.*

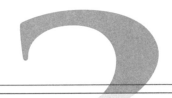

CHAPTER 3
THEORETICAL FRAMEWORK FOR SIMULATION DESIGN
Pamela R. Jeffries, DNS, RN, FAAN, & Kristen J. Rogers, MSN, RN

"If you have knowledge, let others light their
candles at it."

Margaret Fuller

Students' use of patient simulations in nursing education is a relatively efficient method of learning content and critical thinking skills in a safe environment, working collaboratively with the instructor and without fear of causing harm to actual patients (Weis & Guyton-Simmons, 1998). Simulations are defined as activities that mimic reality and variously involve role-playing, interactive videos, or mannequins that help students learn and allow them to demonstrate decision making, critical thinking, and other skills.

Developing, implementing, and evaluating simulations for nursing education can be enhanced by using a framework that specifies relevant variables and their relationships. The need for a consistent and empirically supported model to guide design and implementation and to assess learner outcomes when using simulations has been emphasized by nurse educators as well as leaders in medical education (Cioffi, 2001; Hotchkiss, Biddle, & Fallacaro, 2002). Furthermore, a framework for simulated learning experiences helps scholars conduct research in an organized and systematic fashion rather than in the somewhat haphazard way it has been done to date. When simulation is conducted without benefit of an organizing framework, influencing variables cannot be studied in a consistent way, and educators have difficulty determining the effectiveness of various practices.

The framework presented here was developed based on insights gained from the theoretical and empirical literature related to simulations in nursing, medicine, and other health care disciplines as well as in non-health care disciplines. It was developed for and initially tested through the National League for Nursing/Laerdal Simulation Study (Jeffries, 2005).

The Nursing Education Simulation Framework has five conceptual components (see Figure 3-1), each of which is operationalized through a number of variables. The five concepts include 1) teacher factors, 2) student factors, 3) educational practices that need to be incorporated into the instruction, 4) simulation design characteristics, and 5) expected student outcomes. Each of the components of the framework is discussed in the following sections.

THEORETICAL FRAMEWORK

All instructional strategies, including simulations, should be based on what is known about learning and cognition (Bednar, Cunningham, Duffy, & Perry, 1995), although educators often use an eclectic approach that selects principles and techniques from a variety of theoretical perspectives. For example, collaborative educational learning tools have been based upon behavioral, cognitive information processing, humanistic, and sociocultural theories. Computer-based teaching strategies have drawn upon adult learning, constructivist, and cognitive learning theories.

The Nursing Education Simulation Framework

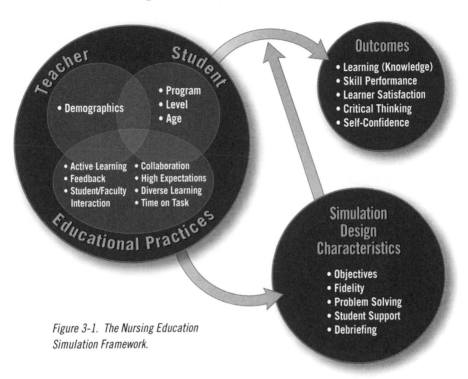

Figure 3-1. The Nursing Education Simulation Framework.

The use of simulations in education has most often been grounded in theories that focus on learner-centered practices, constructivism, and collaboration between individuals with different sociocultural backgrounds. Concepts of learning and cognition (Cunningham, 1996) relevant in designing and using simulations include mind as computer, mind as brain, and mind as rhizome, that is, providing for an infinite number of connections within and outside the sociocultural milieu. These metaphors point to a view of learning as information processing that is respectively a) a cognitive skill; b) experiential growth and pattern recognition; and c) a sociocultural dialogue. When learning is viewed as information processing, instruction is focused on providing efficient communication of information and emphasis is on remembering. When learning is viewed as experiential growth, instruction focuses on experiences and activities that promote the development of cognitive networks and understanding. Finally, when learning is viewed as a sociocultural dialogue, instruction provides opportunities for embedding learning in realistic tasks that lead learners toward participation in a community of practice. Simulations are relevant to each of these perspectives.

FRAMEWORK COMPONENTS

The Teacher

The teacher is essential to the success of any learning experience. However, unlike many traditional classrooms that are teacher-centered, simulations are student-centered, with the teacher playing the roles of facilitator and evaluator. Although other roles have been addressed (Seropian, Brown, Gavilanes, & Driggers, 2004), they are not well developed and are not addressed here.

As a facilitator, the teacher may provide support and encouragement to the learner throughout the simulation, asking questions, proposing "what if" situations, and guiding the debriefing at the conclusion of the experience. As an evaluator, the teacher typically serves strictly as an observer.

Teachers must feel comfortable with and be prepared for the simulations they are using, and they may require assistance with designing the simulation, using the technology, setting up equipment for the activity, and fulfilling the roles of the facilitator and evaluator. In a faculty development workshop where faculty were immersed in a simulation experience, Johnson, Zerwic, and Theis (1999) report that faculty experienced feelings similar to those of students. This activity enabled faculty to identify with students' anxiety and discomforts while participating in this new experience. As part of the simulation framework, selected demographics such as years of experience, age of teacher, and clinical expertise are believed to be associated with the teacher's role, experience, comfort, and overall use of simulations. Further research is needed in this area to explore relationships between selected teacher characteristics and the use of simulations in nursing education.

The Student

Although simulation experiences differ, students generally are expected to be responsible for their own learning; meaning, they need to be self-directed and motivated. Students are more likely to fulfill this responsibility if they know the ground rules for the activity. Such rules encourage and support learning, and acknowledge that mistakes are part of the process. Rules also should minimize competition, which, although a common human motivator, often is detrimental to learning because it may increase anxiety and stress. The ground rules also specify the roles various students will play during the simulation. If the simulation involves group role-playing, the instructor should inform students about the specific role each is to play. Roles vary with the simulation but the most common are patient, nurse, family member, another health care professional, or an unlicensed assistive staff member. In addition, students might also play the role of an observer or recorder. Students may rotate through various roles as the simulation is experienced, and they should discuss each role during the debriefing that follows the experience(s).

Cioffi discusses two types of student roles, response based and process-based, that can be played during a simulation experience. In a response-based role, the learner is not an active participant and has no control over the material presented. An example of this would be assigning a student the role of an observer during the simulation experience. In this role, the student can be part of the simulation but is instructed not to talk, make decisions, or solve problems during the simulation. In a process-based role, the learner is an active participant, making decisions on what information to assess or seek from written resources, the patient and/or family, as well as the sequence and time to seek important information about the client. Examples of this format are patient role-plays, vignettes, and other simulator/simulation activities.

Students also participate in activities designed to judge their progress toward attaining learning outcomes. One such student activity is self-evaluation while viewing a videotape of their performance and using the same critical skills checklist that was used by the faculty during their "live" patient scenario. A study using this approach was reported by Gibbons, Adamo, Padden, Ricciardi, Graziano, Levine, and Hawkins (2002).

As with the teacher concept in the simulation model, the student concept also encompasses variables that may affect the students' simulation experience, performance, and overall learning outcomes when they are involved in a simulation activity. For example, these variables might include the students' age and any experience in nursing care prior to their formal education. More research is needed to explore these variables and others, as well as the impact they have on students and learning outcomes.

Educational Practices

The educational practices component of the simulation framework addresses the features of active learning, diverse learning styles, collaboration, and high expectations. These features need to be considered when designing a simulation in order to improve student performance and satisfaction with their learning (Chickering & Gamson, 1987).

Active learning.

According to Reilly and Oermann (1990), the adult learner will lose interest in an educational experience without active involvement; this engagement in the learning process is critical when designing and using simulations. Active engagement has been shown to enhance students' critical thinking skills (Billings & Halstead, 2005), and it also provides the educator an opportunity to assess the learner's problem-solving and decision-making skills within the context of the simulation experience.

Feedback, an example of active learning with learners, is important to incorporate into any simulation, but whether that feedback should occur during or after the simulation, or both, needs to be thought through carefully. The teacher also needs to decide on the frequency of feedback. Although extensive feedback might be assumed to be helpful, it is important to remember that a simulation should create a safe environment for the learner where mistakes can be made (Henneman & Cunningham, 2005) and where excessive feedback may not be appropriate. If feedback is provided during a simulation, it is important to be careful not to interfere with the learning process. Instead, the learner should be allowed to make a decision, take action, and reflect on that action before feedback is given. Typically, feedback should be given after the simulated experience so the learner has the opportunity to perform and function in the professional role, making decisions and solving problems in the learning situation designed. If instructors provide feedback during the simulation, the student may become dependent upon the instructor for "next steps" or gestures of what to do next.

Diverse learning styles.

According to Dunn and Griggs (1998), understanding that students come to a learning experience with diverse learning styles helps the teacher optimize the learning. Since students might be visual, auditory, tactile, or kinesthetic learners, educators need to incorporate activities into simulations that meet the needs of all learning styles. Fortunately, it is quite easy to do this when designing a simulation, but the degree of emphasis on a learning style will vary depending on the goals and complexity of the simulation.

In the NLN/Laerdal Simulation Study (see Appendix A), strategies were incorporated for all four learning styles. For visual learners, the room was set up to reflect a "real-life" client room; the clock was set to the appropriate time for the beginning of the day shift (7:00 a.m.), and the date was posted on the wall. The auditory learner was accommodated through an audiotaped report from the nurse who had worked the night shift, through SimMan® programming of verbal responses, and through interacting with a student- role-played "family member." The tactile learning style was incorporated though the use of SimMan® because the learner could auscultate lung, bowel, and heart sounds, palpate pulses, and obtain blood pressure readings. Finally, in the client's room, there were dressing supplies, an inspiratory spirometer, and medications, which appealed to the kinesthetic learners because they could actually handle equipment for implementing care.

Collaboration.

According to Billings and Halstead, the student-faculty relationship can influence the learning experience. In order to have a positive impact, the relationship must be collaborative and provide an arena for the exchange of information. This will foster a climate of mutual respect in which the learner feels comfortable asking questions that enhance learning. In developing the simulation, the educator needs to aim for this type of atmosphere. Constructive feedback provided by faculty after the simulation is essential in fostering learning. The educator also needs to obtain feedback about the simulation experience from the learner. This feedback will help the educator to refine the experience. Also, feedback provides an opportunity to address concerns expressed by the learner and promotes active learner involvement in the learning process.

High expectations.

It has been said that when people are expected to do well and they are given the guidance and support needed to succeed, they do succeed. This principle is as relevant for students in a simulation learning experience as it is in other aspects of life. Students should set personal learning goals with faculty and seek advice on how to achieve those goals. When both faculty and students have high expectations for the simulation experience and the outcomes, positive results most often are achieved. Vandrey and Whitman (2001) found that in a safe learning environment using simulations, nurses are able to expand their competency levels and feel empowered to achieve greater learning.

Simulation Design Characteristics

Design characteristics should incorporate five features: objectives, fidelity, problem solving, student support, and reflective thinking (debriefing), all of which must be addressed when developing a simulation. The educator needs to define the features in relation to the simulation purpose and determine the level of inclusion of each feature. The level of inclusion will depend upon the intended outcomes of the simulation.

Objectives.

According to Reilly and Oermann, objectives are the tools that guide learning, and they are essential when using simulations. The objectives of the simulation must reflect the intended outcome of the experience, specify expected learner behaviors, and include sufficient detail to allow the learner to participate in the simulation effectively.

In the NLN/Laerdal Simulation Study (see Appendix A), prior to beginning each experience learners were provided with a list of the purpose and objectives of the simulation. The simulation facilitator read a scripted orientation that provided a brief overview of the different parts of the simulation experience, time frames, students' roles, and a review of the objectives. The objectives were used at the beginning of the simulation to provide direction to learners as they were preparing for the experience.

After the simulation, reference to the objectives can be included in the debriefing, with students explaining how they met the objectives and instructors validating the completion of the objectives.

Fidelity.

Fidelity refers to the extent to which a simulation mimics reality; there are three levels of sophistication (Seropian et al.): high, moderate, and low. High-fidelity simulation incorporates a sophisticated, computerized mannequin that can mimic a real-life situation (e.g., the mannequin's chest rises and falls). In a moderate-fidelity simulation with the mannequin, the chest looks real and breath sounds can be heard, but the chest does not rise and fall. A low-fidelity simulation incorporates static tools (Long, 2005) (e.g., a mannequin with no extra features such as breath and heart sounds, voice, or any interactive features).

If the purpose of the simulation is skill attainment, (e.g., IM injection), then a low-fidelity simulation, such as an injection pad and a syringe, is sufficient. If the purpose of the experience is to enhance the students' critical thinking skills in caring for clients with end-stage kidney disease, a high-fidelity simulation would provide a "close-to-life" situation that allows for patient-nurse communication and exhibition of appropriate signs and symptoms.

In developing a high-fidelity simulation, the real-life situation must be replicated as closely as possible (Medley & Horne, 2005). In the NLN/Laerdal Simulation Study (see Appendix A), for example, this was done by programming a patient simulator (SimMan®) with selected verbal responses, creating a post-operative incision, setting up the room with medications and supplies, having a student portray a family member, and providing an audiotaped client report.

Problem solving.

Problem solving is related to the level of complexity of the simulation, which in turn needs to be based on the knowledge and skill level of the learners. The educator needs to reflect on the purpose of the experience and the learner's abilities when determining the level of complexity. A complex simulation should be at a level that is challenging to the learner but attainable. If the level is unattainable, the simulation will not be an effective learning experience for the learner. Although it is important to try to mimic a real-life situation, it is important not to overload the learner with too much information just because the simulator has a variety of options (Rauen, 2001). In a complex simulation, the educator wants to provide the learner an opportunity to prioritize nursing assessments and provide care based on the assessments, then be able to perform a self-evaluation.

Student support.

The support feature focuses on the assistance provided to the student. In creating the simulation, the educator needs to determine how and when support and assistance will be provided by the facilitator: a cue from another individual involved in the simulation, a lab report, a phone call, or another type of cueing mechanism. Assistance should be in the form of cues that offer enough information for the learner to continue with the simulation but do not interfere with his/her independent problem solving. For example, if the student is performing a head-to-toe assessment and the patient begins to experience chest tightness, the student may be so focused on the assessment that she ignores the complaint of chest tightness. The educator can provide cues through programming the patient simulator to verbalize the pain or instructing the "family" ahead of time to ask if the nurse could do something about the patient's pain if necessary, as it is not like him to complain. Cues like this alert the nurse to the patient's pain and, it is hoped, direct the assessments and attention to this patient problem.

Reflective thinking/debriefing.

Immediately following the simulation experience, students and faculty engage in a debriefing in which they examine what happened and what was learned. This reflective thinking session (Henneman & Cunningham) provides learners with an opportunity to assess their actions, decisions, communications, and ability to deal with the unexpected in the simulation. This session should occur immediately after the simulation is completed so the thoughts and feelings of the learner are not forgotten and do not get distorted over time.

The reflective thinking session needs to be guided by the educator so remarks focus on the learning outcomes and the application of learned concepts to practice (Rauen). Discussion often is enhanced if the educator develops specific topics for discussion that are related to the objectives. For example, to prioritize nursing concerns for the client, the discussion would focus on constructive comments and learning instead of criticism (Medley & Horne). Table 3-1 lists the questions used during the reflective thinking session of the NLN/Laerdal Simulation Study (see Appendix A). These questions evolved from the objectives of the simulation experience and helped the educator assess how well they had been met. The questions also helped the educator clarify any misperceptions, correct any errors that had been made, and emphasize correct, appropriate, and safe nursing care and decision making.

Table 3-1. Reflective Thinking/Debriefing Questions

1. How did you feel throughout the simulation experience?

2. Describe the objectives you were able to achieve.

3. Which ones were you unable to achieve (if any)?

4. Did you have the knowledge and skills to meet objectives?

5. Were you satisfied with your ability to work through the situation?

6. To Observer: Could the nurses have handled any aspects of the simulation differently?

7. If you were able to do this again, how could you have handled the situation differently?

8. What did the group do well?

9. What did the team think was the primary nursing diagnosis?

10. What were the key assessments and interventions?

11. Is there anything else you would like to discuss?

Reflective Thinking Session Guidelines

1. The person who conducts the reflective thinking must observe the simulation.

2. Immediately after the simulation, the students are taken away from the bedside to a separate room for guided reflection.

3. The guided reflection session should last 20 minutes: 10 minutes for discussing content; 10 minutes for reflective thinking.

4. The facilitator doing the debriefing should correct and discuss any inappropriate actions that occurred, missed assessments, or interventions.

5. If time runs out and students still want to discuss the event, direct them to use reflective journaling and turn in to the instructor.

6. Give a 5 minute warning before the end of the simulation itself and before the end of reflective thinking session.

Outcomes

The final component of the Simulation Framework (see Figure 3-1) is outcomes, such as knowledge gained, skills performed, learners' satisfaction, critical thinking, and self-confidence. As noted, learning outcomes need to be established and discussed prior to the simulation. In addition, the approaches and tools used to measure attainment of the objectives must be established in advance. Evaluating outcomes is essential to determining what students have learned and the overall effectiveness of the simulation experience

(Kirkpatrick, DeWitt-Weaver, & Yeager, 2005). The nurse educator might want to ask the following questions to evaluate the simulation experience:

- Did it provide the type of experience desired by the instructor and students?
- Was it an effective use of faculty time and resources?
- Were there problems or concerns with the implementation phase of the simulation?
- Did the simulation produce the preestablished outcomes?
- What revisions are necessary?
- Are appropriate evaluation methods being used to assess the outcomes needed?
- Did students learn the objectives outlined for the simulation?
- Did the simulation provide the learning outcomes expected for learners?

Summary

A framework that identifies significant components of simulations and the relationships among these components is a very useful guide to the design, implementation, and evaluation of simulation activities. Simulations for teaching and learning are complex, multifaceted, and challenging. It is hoped that the use of the framework described here will enhance the development, implementation, and evaluation of this exciting and innovative teaching/learning strategy in nursing education. With continued use and testing of the simulation framework, components of and interrelationships within the framework will evolve and improve over time.

REFERENCES

Bednar, A., Cunningham, D. J., Duffy, T., & Perry, D. (1995). Theory into practice: How do we link? In G. Anglin (Ed.), _Instructional technology: Past, present, and future_ (2nd ed.) (pp. 100-112). Englewood, CO: Libraries Unlimited.

Billings, D. M., & Halstead, J. A. (2005). _Teaching in nursing: A guide for faculty_ (2nd ed.). Philadelphia: W. B. Saunders.

Chickering, A. W., & Gamson, Z. F. (1987, March). Seven principles of good practice in undergraduate education. _AAHE Bulletin, 39_(7), 5-10.

Cioffi, J. (2001). Clinical simulations: Development and validation. _Nurse Education Today, 21_, 477-486.

Cunningham, D. (1996). Time after time. In W. Spinks (Ed.), _Semiotics 95_ (pp. 263-269). New York: Lang.

Dunn, R., & Griggs, S.A. (1998). _Learning styles and the nursing profession_. New York: NLN Press.

Gibbons, S., Adamo, G., Padden, D., Ricciardi, R., Graziano, M., Levine, E., & Hawkins, R. (2002). Clinical evaluation in advanced practice nursing education: Using standardized patients in health assessment. _Journal of Nursing Education, 41_(5), 215-221.

Henneman, E. A., & Cunningham, H. (2005). Using clinical simulation to teach patient safety in an acute/critical care nursing course. _Nurse Educator, 30_(4), 172-177.

Hotchkiss, M., Biddle, C., & Fallacaro, M. (2002). Assessing the authenticity of the human simulation experience in anesthesiology. _AANA Journal, 70_(6), 470-473.

Jeffries, P. R. (2005). A framework for designing, implementing, and evaluating simulations used as teaching strategies in nursing. _Nursing Education Perspectives, 26_(2), 96-103.

Johnson, J. H., Zerwic, J. J., & Theis, S. L. (1999). Clinical simulation laboratory: An adjunct to clinical teaching. _Nurse Educator, 24_(5), 37-41.

Kirkpatrick, J., DeWitt-Weaver, D., & Yeager, L. (2005). Strategies for evaluating learning outcomes. In D. Billings, & J. Halstead (Eds.), _Teaching in nursing: A guide for faculty_ (2nd ed.) (pp. 367-384). Philadelphia: W. B. Saunders.

Long, R.E. (2005). Using simulation to teach resuscitation: An important patient safety tool. _Critical Care Nursing Clinics of North America, 17_(1), 1-8.

Medley, C. F. & Horne, C. (2005). Using simulation technology for undergraduate nursing education. *Journal of Nursing Education, 44*(1), 31-34.

Rauen, C. A. (2001). Using simulation to teach critical thinking skills. *Critical Care Nursing Clinics of North America, 13*(1), 93-103.

Reilly, D. E. & Oermann, M. (1990). *Behavioral objectives: Evaluation in nursing* (3rd ed.). New York: National League for Nursing.

Seropian, M. A., Brown, K., Gavilanes, J. S., & Driggers, B. (2004). Simulation: Not just a manikin. *Journal of Nursing Education, 43*(4), 164-169.

Vandrey, C., & Whitman, M. (2001). Simulator training for novice critical care nurses. *American Journal of Nursing, 101*(9), 24GG-24LL.

Weis, P., & Guyton-Simmons, J. (1998). A computer simulation for teaching critical thinking skills. *Nurse Educator, 23*(2), 30-33.

CHAPTER 4

DESIGNING SIMULATIONS FOR NURSING EDUCATION

Janis C. Childs, PhD, RN, Susan B. Sepples, PhD, CCRN, & Kristy Chambers, MSN, RN

"Good teaching is one-fourth preparation
and three-fourths theatre."

Gail Godwin

With the simulation framework reviewed and described in detail, the next step is to use the framework to develop your own simulations. This chapter highlights important concepts, relates the design of a simulation to the nursing process, and provides a template for creating your own curriculum-specific scenarios. In addition, a completed template that can be used as an example is provided to assist you in getting started.

Simulation design and development often are thought to be so time-consuming that faculty simply do not have the resources or support to integrate simulation into their courses. It is true that since this teaching strategy is new to many, it requires heightened attention initially, as is the case when doing anything new. However, research documents that taking the time to create realistic simulations "pays off" for students and faculty alike (Beyea & Kobokovich, 2004; Childs & Sepples, 2006; McCausland, Curran, & Cataldi, 2004), so it appears to be a worthwhile investment. Also, the more one designs simulations the easier and more satisfying the process becomes. As one becomes more comfortable with simulation design, learning experiences of varying depth and complexity can be created so that simulations can be used effectively with beginning students, advanced students, and professionals.

Students report being more excited about learning, learning more, gaining confidence in their skills, and actually looking forward to learning when well-crafted simulations are utilized. Faculty report satisfaction with this teaching strategy and indicate a renewed excitement about their teaching role. Finally, both faculty and students report being more engaged with each other when simulation is used. In light of these documented benefits, faculty would do well to learn how to design educationally-sound simulation scenarios.

Faculty can draw on their clinical experience and theoretical expertise when creating simulations to facilitate student learning, and they can be highly innovative. Indeed, the only limitation in creating a simulation is one's own lack of imagination (Medley & Horne, 2005; Seropian, Brown, Gavilanes & Driggers, 2004).

Before getting started, review the simulation framework presented in chapter 3 of this text, as it will help to you to create a simulation that is appropriate for you, your students, and your curriculum. In essence, the components that are important to include in a simulation are as follows:

Best practices in education that provide for active learning, provide feedback, incorporate student-faculty interactions, provide for collaborative learning, set high expectations, attend to the needs of diverse learners, and provide for appropriate time on task

Student factors, such as designating specific roles for students and allowing for self-directed learning

Faculty factors, such as determining the appropriate use of support/cues and allowing for an observer/evaluator

Simulation design characteristics that clarify learning objectives, provide fidelity within the simulation, determine the appropriate level of complexity, imbed cues, and provide adequate debriefing opportunities

Outcomes that include knowledge, skill performance, learner satisfaction, critical thinking, and self-confidence

USING THE NURSING PROCESS TO GUIDE SIMULATION DESIGN

The nursing process remains a relevant and widely utilized guide to getting started with the planning and design of a simulation that will be appropriate for your course or unit of study. While keeping the simulation framework in mind, consider using the nursing process as follows:

Assessment ... Assess your school's curriculum, concentrating on how and where simulation might work to the best advantage of students and faculty. Identify program strengths and limitations and determine where simulation might build on those strengths or improve on any areas of limitation. Determine how simulation experiences will help students achieve overall objectives and how they can be used to evaluate student learning, alone or in combination with other evaluation methods.

Diagnosis ... After gathering data about your program, determine where simulation might fit best, and whether it will further support areas that are strengths or strengthen areas that are weak. For simulation to be successful, it must be carefully planned and incorporated into the curriculum where it will be most effective and viable. Identifying faculty who are ready to engage and learn the benefit of integrating simulation into their courses also is a key factor in the success of increased use of simulations.

Planning ... Create a case study that incorporates the learning outcomes that faculty want students to achieve or that will be the basis for evaluating students. Use this case study to create a scenario that will guide the simulation experience. The template provided in Figure 4-1 can be used as a guide and adapted to accommodate outcomes that are relevant and specific to your case study. Figure 4-2 provides an example of a completed simulation design for care of a post-operative adult patient. You will see how the basic template (Figure 4-1) has been used to create a scenario that can be used to guide learning. Students are provided with learning objectives, background information on the patient, lab values, and other pertinent information; lab staff are provided with information that will help them organize and set up the scenario; and faculty or professional staff who will run the scenario and conduct the debriefing session are provided with information that help them implement those roles. In essence, it is critical that faculty plan all the details of the simulation in advance in order to ensure a successful learning experience.

Implementation ... Once the simulation is carefully and thoroughly planned, gather all the items that will be needed to mimic reality and enhance student success. This is where imagination will come into play. Simulations that replicate the practice area as closely as possible are the experiences that are most valuable. Perform a "practice" simulation with faculty colleagues and/or students in order to identify difficulties or adaptations that might need to be made prior to actually using the simulation with learners. This is an indispensable step in creating a successful experience.

Evaluation ... Following the experience, ask questions such as these: In general, how did it go? Did students meet the objectives? How did the students perform during the simulation? How well did students and faculty work together? Did anything hinder the progress of the simulation? Were there problems with the technology? Answers to these and other questions will guide you in making changes for when you use the scenario again.

MAKING THE MOST OF THE SIMULATION DESIGN TEMPLATE

Background and Context

The templates provided as Figures 4-1 and 4-2 are useful in helping faculty get started in designing a simulation experience; however, they are not intended to be followed without modification. For example, if your program focuses on family-centered care and the simulation is intended to help students learn how to incorporate this concept into practice, the learning objectives can be written to focus more on this aspect than on others, family care can be highlighted in the readings, and more family roles can be assigned. Such variations can provide a rich learning experience for students and help them enhance their ability to provide family-centered care in the clinical setting.

Incorporated into the simulation design template is a listing of the NCLEX-RN® categories and sub-categories. This can help you create a scenario that emphasizes those concepts faculty wish to address, and an examination of all scenarios used throughout your students' educational experience can help faculty determine which concepts receive extensive attention and which are touched upon only minimally. Such an analysis can help faculty evaluate the curriculum, propose revisions that are based on data, and enhance student learning and, perhaps, success on the licensing exam.

Roles

Simulation allows for individuals to assume the role of patient, health care provider, family member, or other individual. Students might be assigned to assume these roles, or members of the community might be invited to participate in the simulation experience. Community members, including nurses from clinical facilities where your students affiliate, might participate in the planning or in the actual simulation experience with students. In addition, if your institution offers programs in medicine, pharmacy social work or other health care professions, you might consult with faculty in those fields about writing case studies or involving their students in the scenario. Whatever the approach selected, designing and implementing simulations provide an excellent opportunity for collaboration within your institution and community.

Simulation also provides opportunities for students to work with people from diverse backgrounds. Many mannequins can be programmed to provide information about the patient's culture, religion, gender, or sexuality as well as physiologic functioning; or students themselves can assume roles of individuals with diverse backgrounds. You might design an experience that requires students to work with a language translator or a translator for the hearing impaired. If your institution offers classes in sign language, you might involve a student teaching the patient and his family how to perform a skill (e.g., wound care).

Whatever the role that is to be enacted, it is critical that you write a brief synopsis of the role, including what the person assuming it might be expected to say or do. Such a synopsis helps move the simulation along and ensures that important concepts and learning objectives are achieved.

Technology/Equipment

Understanding and knowing your resources as well as your own strengths and limitations to conduct simulation experiences are paramount. If you have a high-fidelity simulator, you must have a working knowledge of the technology, but you do not have to be an expert to get started!

For the most part, there are three ways that you can "run" a simulation with a high-fidelity mannequin: manual mode, manual mode with trends, and preprogrammed. The **manual mode** often is referred to as operating a scenario "on the fly" since the person at the computer makes changes depending on student responses and actions; nothing is pre-programmed. The **manual mode with trends** allows for some "on the fly" changing and adaptation to the scenario as students work through the case study, but it also contains some preprogrammed responses or trends. **Preprogrammed** scenarios come with the mannequin, are available from the manufacturer, or are created by faculty; they direct what happens and when in response to students' actions.

How you utilize a high-fidelity simulator will vary depending on your comfort with the technology, your personal preferences, the objectives for the experience, and whether you are using simulation for a teaching-learning experience or for evaluation. Do not be discouraged, as the more you utilize the high-fidelity mannequins, the more comfortable you will feel. This comfort will allow you to create case studies and experiences that are more and more complex and stimulating for faculty and students.

Guided Reflection

Guided reflection is an essential aspect of a simulation experience. Chapter 6 is dedicated to this important learning tool as a part of the overall simulation experience, so you might want to review it for more detail. Several "standard" guided reflection questions are included with the templates provided as Figures 4-1 and 4-2 so you can see how they must be thought about as part of the planning phase. Questions posed during the guided reflection session will, of course, need to be relevant to the learning objectives for the simulation, significant curricular threads, and special points you want to emphasize with students.

SUMMARY

This chapter provides a template to guide faculty in designing simulations that will enhance student learning. It also provides an example that serves to illustrate how the template can be used to plan an effective scenario. Both resources, along with the "helpful hints" provided, are intended to help faculty as they begin the journey of incorporating simulation into courses and the overall curriculum.

It is important to remember that the careful and thoughtful design of a simulation is a key factor in determining its success or failure. But once that time and energy are invested, the simulation is implemented and evaluated, and student learning outcomes are assessed, faculty are well on their way to creating more exciting, relevant simulations that can meet the learning needs of diverse learners.

REFERENCES

Beyea, S. C., & Kobokovich, L. J., (2004). Human patient simulations: A teaching strategy. _Association of Operating Room Nurses, 80_(4), 738-742.

Childs, J. C., & Sepples, S. B. (2006). Clinical teaching by simulation: Lessons learned from a complex patient care scenario. _Nursing Education Perspectives, 27_(3), 154-158.

McCausland, L. L., Curran, C. C., & Cataldi, P. (2004). Use of a human simulator for undergraduate nurse education. _International Journal of Nursing Education Scholarship, 1_(1), 1-17.

Medley, C. F., & Horne, C. (2005). Using simulation technology for undergraduate nursing education. _Journal of Nursing Education, 44_(1), 31-34.

Seropian, M. A., Brown, K., Gavilanes, J. S., & Driggers, B. (2004). Simulation: Not just a manikin. _Journal of Nursing Education, 43_(4), 164-169.

FIGURE 4-1. SIMULATION DESIGN TEMPLATE

Simulation Design Template

Scenario File:

Discipline: _____   Student Level: _____

Expected Simulation Run Time: _____   Guided Reflection Time: _____

Location: _____   Location for Reflection: _____

Admission Date: Today's Date:	**Psychomotor Skills Required Prior to Simulation**
Brief Description of Client	
Name:	
Gender: Age:	
Race:	
Weight: ____kg Height: ____cm	
Religion: Major Support:	
Phone:	
Allergies:	
Immunizations:	**Cognitive Activities Required Prior to Simulation**
	[i.e. independent reading (R), video review (V),
Attending Physician/Team:	*computer simulations (CS), lecture (L)]*
Past Medical History:	
History of Present illness:	
Social History:	**Nursing Diagnosis:**
Primary Medical Diagnosis:	
Surgeries/Procedures & Dates:	

Simulation Learning Objectives

1.

2.

3.

4.

5.

6.

7.

8.

Scenario Specific Objectives

Program / Curriculum Specific Objectives

Fidelity (choose all that apply to this simulation)

Setting/Environment
- ❏ ER
- ❏ Med Surg
- ❏ Peds
- ❏ ICU
- ❏ OR / PACU
- ❏ Women's Center
- ❏ Behavioral Health
- ❏ Home Health
- ❏ Pre-Hospital
- ❏ Other _____

Simulator/Mannequin/s Needed:

Props:

Equipment Attached to Mannequin:
- ❏ IV tubing with primary line ____fluids running at ____cc/hr
- ❏ Secondary IV line ___ running at ___ cc/hr
- ❏ IV pump
- ❏ Foley catheter _____cc output
- ❏ PCA pump running
- ❏ IVPB with ___ running at ___ cc/hr
- ❏ 02 _____
- ❏ Monitor attached
- ❏ ID band
- ❏ Other _____

Equipment Available in Room
- ❏ Bedpan/Urinal
- ❏ Foley kit
- ❏ Straight Cath Kit
- ❏ Incentive Spirometry
- ❏ Fluids
- ❏ IV start kit
- ❏ IV tubing
- ❏ IVPB Tubing
- ❏ IV Pump
- ❏ Feeding Pump
- ❏ Pressure Bag
- ❏ 02 delivery device_____
- ❏ Crash cart with airway devices and emergency medications
- ❏ Defibrillator/Pacer
- ❏ Suction
- ❏ Other

Medications and Fluids
- ❏ Oral Meds
- ❏ IV Fluids
- ❏ IVPB
- ❏ IV Push
- ❏ IM / Subcut / Intradermal
- ❏ Other_____

Diagnostics Available
- ❏ X-rays (Images)
- ❏ Labs
- ❏ 12-Lead EKG
- ❏ Other_____

Documentation Forms
- ❏ Admit Orders
- ❏ Physician Orders
- ❏ Flow sheet
- ❏ Medication Administration Record
- ❏ Kardex
- ❏ Graphic Record
- ❏ Shift Assessment
- ❏ Triage Forms
- ❏ Code Record
- ❏ Anesthesia / PACU Record
- ❏ Standing (Protocol) Orders
- ❏ Transfer Orders
- ❏ Other

**Recommended Mode for Simulation
(i.e. manual, programmed, etc.)**

Fidelity (con't.)

Roles/Guidelines for Roles
- ❏ Primary Nurse
- ❏ Secondary Nurse
- ❏ Clinical Instructor
- ❏ Family Member #1
- ❏ Family Member #2
- ❏ Observer
- ❏ Physician / Advanced Practice Nurse
- ❏ Respiratory Therapy
- ❏ Anesthesia
- ❏ Pharmacy
- ❏ Lab
- ❏ Imaging
- ❏ Social Services
- ❏ Clergy
- ❏ Unlicensed Assistive Personnel
- ❏ Code Team
- ❏ Other_____

Important Information Related to Roles

Significant Lab Values

Physician Orders

Student Information Needed Prior to Scenario
- ❏ Has been oriented to simulator
- ❏ Understands guidelines /expectations for scenario
- ❏ Has accomplished all pre-simulation requirements
- ❏ All participants understand their assigned roles
- ❏ Has been given time frame expectations
- ❏ Other _____

Report Students Will Receive Before Simulation

Time:

References, Evidence-Based Practice Guidelines, Protocols,
or Algorithms Used For This Scenario: (site source, author, year, and page)

2007 NCLEX-RN® Test Plan Categories and Subcategories

Choose all areas included in the simulation

Safe and Effective Care Environment

Management of Care
- ❏ Advance Directives
- ❏ Advocacy
- ❏ Case Management
- ❏ Client Rights
- ❏ Collaboration with Interdisciplinary Team
- ❏ Concepts of Management
- ❏ Confidentiality / Information Security
- ❏ Consultation
- ❏ Continuity of Care
- ❏ Delegation
- ❏ Establishing Priorities
- ❏ Ethical Practice
- ❏ Informed Consent
- ❏ Information Technology
- ❏ Legal Rights and Responsibilities
- ❏ Performance Improvement (QI)
- ❏ Referrals
- ❏ Resource Management
- ❏ Staff Education
- ❏ Supervision

Safety and Infection Control
- ❏ Accident Prevention
- ❏ Disaster Planning
- ❏ Emergency Response Plan
- ❏ Ergonomic Response Plan
- ❏ Error Prevention
- ❏ Handling Hazardous and Infectious Materials
- ❏ Home Safety
- ❏ Injury Prevention
- ❏ Medical and Surgical Asepsis
- ❏ Reporting of Incident/Event/
- ❏ Irregular Occurrence/Variance
- ❏ Security Plan
- ❏ Standard /Transmission-Based/ Other Precautions
- ❏ Use of Restraints/Safety Devices
- ❏ Safe Use of Equipment

Health Promotion and Maintenance

- ❏ Aging Process
- ❏ Ante/Intra/Postpartum and Newborn Care
- ❏ Developmental Stages and Transitions
- ❏ Disease Prevention
- ❏ Expected Body Image Changes
- ❏ Family Planning
- ❏ Family Systems
- ❏ Growth and Development
- ❏ Health and Wellness
- ❏ Health Promotion Programs
- ❏ Health Screening
- ❏ High Risk Behaviors
- ❏ Human Sexuality
- ❏ Immunizations
- ❏ Lifestyle Choices
- ❏ Principles of Teaching/Learning
- ❏ Self-Care
- ❏ Techniques of Physical Assessment

Psychosocial Integrity

- ❏ Abuse/Neglect
- ❏ Behavioral Interventions
- ❏ Chemical and Other Dependencies
- ❏ Coping Mechanisms
- ❏ Crisis Intervention
- ❏ Cultural Diversity
- ❏ End of Life Care
- ❏ Family Dynamics
- ❏ Grief and Loss
- ❏ Mental Health Concepts
- ❏ Psychopathology
- ❏ Religious and Spiritual Influences on Health
- ❏ Sensory/Perceptual Alterations
- ❏ Situational Role Changes
- ❏ Stress Management
- ❏ Support Systems
- ❏ Therapeutic Communications
- ❏ Therapeutic Environment
- ❏ Unexpected Body Image Changes

2007 NCLEX-RN® Test Plan Categories and Subcategories (Con.t)
Choose all areas included in the simulation

Physiologic Integrity
Basic Care and Comfort
- ❑ Assistive Devices
- ❑ Complementary and Alternative Therapies
- ❑ Elimination
- ❑ Mobility/Immobility
- ❑ Non-Pharmacological Comfort Interventions
- ❑ Nutrition and Oral Hydration
- ❑ Palliative/Comfort Care
- ❑ Personal Hygiene
- ❑ Rest and Sleep

Pharmacological and Parenteral Therapies
- ❑ Adverse Effects/Contraindications
- ❑ Blood and Blood Products
- ❑ Central Venous Access Devices
- ❑ Dosage Calculation
- ❑ Expected Effects/Outcomes
- ❑ Medication Administration
- ❑ Parenteral/Intravenous Therapies
- ❑ Pharmacological Agents/Actions
- ❑ Pharmacological Interactions
- ❑ Pharmacological Pain Management
- ❑ Total Parenteral Nutrition

Reduction of Risk Potential
- ❑ Diagnostic Tests
- ❑ Lab Values
- ❑ Monitoring Conscious Sedation
- ❑ Potential for Alterations in Body Systems
- ❑ Potential for Complications of Diagnostic Tests/Treatments/Procedures
- ❑ Potential for Complications from Surgical Procedures and Health Alterations
- ❑ System Specific Assessments
- ❑ Therapeutic Procedures
- ❑ Vital Signs

Physiologic Adaptation
- ❑ Alterations in Body Systems
- ❑ Fluid and Electrolyte Imbalances
- ❑ Hemodynamics
- ❑ Illness Management
- ❑ Infectious Diseases
- ❑ Medical Emergencies
- ❑ Pathophysiology
- ❑ Radiation Therapy
- ❑ Unexpected Response to Therapies

Scenario Progression Outline

Timing (Approximate)	Mannequin Actions	Expected Interventions	May Use the Following Cues
First 5 minutes			Role member providing cue: Cue:
Next 5-10 minutes			Role member providing cue: Cue:
Final 15-20 minutes			Role member providing cue: Cue:

Debriefing / Guided Reflection Questions for this Simulation

(Remember to identify important concepts or curricular threads that are specific to your program)

1.
2.
3.
4.
5.
6.
7.
8.
9.
10.
11.

Scenario Specific Questions:

Program/Curricular Specific Questions:

Complexity – Simple to Complex

Suggestions for changing the complexity of this scenario to adapt to different levels of learners:

•
•
•

FIGURE 4-2. CARE OF A POST-OPERATIVE ADULT PATIENT: SIMULATION DESIGN

Patient Care Simulation

Scenario File: Basic Postoperative Care (Vernon Watkins)
Discipline: Nursing   Student Level: Fundamentals/Basic
Expected Simulation Run Time: 20 Minutes   Guided Reflection Time: 20 Minutes

Admission Date: 5/26 **Today's Date:** 5/29	**Psychomotor Skills Required Prior to Simulation**
Brief Description of Client:	
Name: Vernon Watkins	- Basic assessment skills
Gender: M **Age:** 69	- Receiving report
Race: Caucasian	- Taking vital signs
Weight: 77 kg **Height:** 180 cm	- Incentive spirometry
Religion: Not Stated	- Wound assessment and dressing change
Major Support: Wife	- Medication administration
Phone: 720-0000	- IV maintenance
	- Recording intake and output
Allergies:	
Peniciliin (hives)	
Immunizations:	**Cognitive Activities Required Prior to Simulation**
current, gets flu shot every year	*[i.e. independent reading (R), video review (V), computer simulations (CS), lecture (L)]*
Attending Physician/Team:	
Dr. CT Sniff	- Care of the Postoperative Patient
Past Medical History:	- Wound Management
History of cataracts, controlled hypertension, smokes ½ pack filtered cigarettes/day, walks 3 miles/day.	- Safe Medication Administration - Patient teaching regarding use of incentive spirometry
History of Present illness:	
Presented to ER 5/26 with complaints of nausea, vomiting, and severe abdominal pain. Admitted for emergent surgery for bowel perforation.	**Nursing Diagnosis:** - Acute Pain - Risk for Impaired Gas Exchange
Social History:	- Risk for Ineffective Airway Clearance
Retired postal service worker, enjoys yard work.	- Impaired Physical Mobility - Risk for Thrombophlebitis
Primary Medical Diagnosis:	
Perforated Colon	
Surgeries/Procedures & Dates:	
Hemicolectomy 5/26	

Simulation Learning Objectives

1. Apply the nursing process to initiate care of the postoperative patient.

2. Assess the postoperative patient, including information obtained through communication.

3. Determine (plan) the nursing care for the patient based on assessment findings.

4. Implement the appropriate care in a safe manner.

5. Evaluate the care provided.

6. Identify the primary nursing diagnosis and/or collaborative problems.

7. Document the assessments, patient changes, and interventions completed.

8. Demonstrate therapeutic communications in care of the patient and family.

Fidelity (choose all that apply to this simulation)

Setting/Environment
- ❏ ER
- ☑ Med Surg - bed, with chair for wife at bedside, overbed table
- ❏ Peds
- ❏ ICU
- ❏ OR / PACU
- ❏ Women's Center
- ❏ Behavioral Health
- ❏ Home Health
- ❏ Pre-Hospital
- ❏ Other _____

Simulator/Mannequin/s Needed: SimMan

Props: SimMan in hospital gown

Equipment Attached to Mannequin:
- ☑ IV tubing with primary line <u>D5W</u> fluids running at <u>100</u> cc/hr
- ❏ Secondary IV line ___ running at ___ cc/hr
- ❏ IV pump
- ❏ Foley catheter _____cc output
- ❏ PCA pump running
- ❏ IVPB with ___ running at ___ cc/hr
- ❏ 02 _____
- ❏ Monitor attached
- ☑ ID band - Watkins, Vernon # 529-52-6
- ☑ Other - abdominal wound with 4x4 dressing applied - small amount of blood on dressing

Equipment Available in Room
- ❏ Bedpan/Urinal
- ❏ Foley kit
- ☑ Straight Catheter Kit
- ☑ Incentive Spirometry
- ❏ Fluids
- ❏ IV start kit
- ❏ IV tubing
- ❏ IVPB Tubing
- ❏ IV Pump
- ❏ Feeding Pump
- ❏ Pressure Bag
- ☑ 02 delivery device
- ❏ Crash cart with airway devices and emergency medications
- ❏ Defibrillator/Pacer
- ❏ Suction
- ☑ Other - Sterile 2x2, sterile 4x4, sterile fields, ABD pads, 1" and 2" tape, bottle of NSS, sterile gloves, exam gloves

Medications and Fluids
- ☑ Oral Meds:
  - Zantac (ranitidine) 75 mg PO TID
  - Fe Sulfate 324 mg PO TID before meals
  - Percocet (oxycodone/acetaminophen) 1-2 PO every 4 hours PRN
  - Tylenol (acetaminophen) 2 PO every 4 hours PRN for headache
- ☑ IV Fluids: 1 liter D5W at 100ml/hr followed by 1 liter 5% dextrose / 0.45 NaCl at 80ml/hr
- ☑ IVPB: Ancef 1 gram IVPB every 8 hours (to infuse over 30 minutes
- ❏ IV Push
- ❏ IM / Subcut / Intradermal
- ❏ Other_____

Diagnostics Available
- ❏ X-rays (Images)
- ☑ Labs
- ❏ 12-Lead EKG
- ❏ Other_____

Documentation Forms
- ❏ Admit Orders
- ☑ Physician Orders
- ☑ Flow sheet
- ☑ Medication Administration Record
- ☑ Kardex
- ☑ Graphic Record
- ☑ Shift Assessment
- ❏ Triage Forms
- ❏ Code Record
- ❏ Anesthesia / PACU Record
- ❏ Standing (Protocol) Orders
- ❏ Transfer Orders
- ☑ Other: signature sheet, 24 hour Intake and Output Sheet, Braden Scale, Progress Notes

Recommended Mode for Simulation
(i.e. manual, programmed, etc.)

This is a preprogrammed scenario with prerecorded vocal sounds.

References, Evidence-Based Practice Guidelines, Protocols, or Algorithms Used For This Scenario: (site source, author, year, and page)

During the first 24 hours after surgery, nursing care of the hospitalized patient on the general medical-surgical unit involves continuing to help the patient recover from the effects of anesthesia, frequently assessing the patient's physiologic status, monitoring complications, managing pain, and implementing measures designed to achieve the long-range goals of independence with self-care, successful management of the thera-peutic regimen, discharge to home, and full recovery. Postoperative patient's are at risk for complications such as atelectasis, pneumonia, deep vein thrombosis, pulmonary embolism, constipation, paralytic ilius, and wound infection.

Respiratory depressive effects of opioid medications, decreased lung expansion secondary to pain, and decreased mobility combine to put the patient at risk for common respiratory complications, particularly atelectasis. Signs and symptoms include decreased breath sounds, crackles, and cough.

Preventative measures and timely recognition of signs and symptoms help avert pulmonary complications. Strategies to prevent respiratory complications include use of an incentive spirometer and deep breathing and coughing exercises.

After major abdominal surgery, distention may be avoided by having the patient turn frequently, exercise, and ambulate as early as possible. The nurse can determine when peristaltic bowel sounds return by listening to the abdomen with a stethoscope. Bowel sounds are documented so that diet progression can occur.

Reference
Institute for Safe Medication Practices website: http://www.ismp.org

NANDA International (Ed.). (2005). NANDA nursing diagnosis: Definitions and classification. Philadelphia: Author.

Smeltzer, S.C., & Bare, B.G. (2004). Postoperative nursing management. In R. Hallowell & T. Gibbons (Eds.), Brunner & Suddarth's textbook of medical-surgical nursing (10th ed.) (pp. 445-453). Philadelphia, PA: Lippincott Williams and Wilkins.

2007 NCLEX-RN® Test Plan Categories and Subcategories
Choose all areas included in the simulation

Safe and Effective Care Environment
Management of Care
- ❏ Advance Directives
- ❏ Advocacy
- ❏ Case Management
- ❏ Client Rights
- ❏ Collaboration with Interdisciplinary Team
- ❏ Concepts of Management
- ❏ Confidentiality / Information Security
- ❏ Consultation
- ❏ Continuity of Care
- ☑ Delegation
- ☑ Establishing Priorities
- ❏ Ethical Practice
- ❏ Informed Consent
- ❏ Information Technology
- ❏ Legal Rights and Responsibilities
- ❏ Performance Improvement (QI)
- ❏ Referrals
- ❏ Resource Management
- ❏ Staff Education
- ❏ Supervision

Safety and Infection Control
- ❏ Accident Prevention
- ❏ Disaster Planning
- ❏ Emergency Response Plan
- ❏ Ergonomic Response Plan
- ❏ Error Prevention
- ❏ Handling Hazardous and Infectious Materials
- ❏ Home Safety
- ❏ Injury Prevention
- ☑ Medical and Surgical Asepsis
- ❏ Reporting of Incident/Event/
- ❏ Irregular Occurrence/Variance
- ❏ Security Plan
- ☑ Standard /Transmission-Based / Other Precautions
- ❏ Use of Restraints/Safety Devices
- ❏ Safe Use of Equipment

Health Promotion and Maintenance
- ❏ Aging Process
- ❏ Ante/Intra/Postpartum and Newborn Care
- ❏ Developmental Stages and Transitions
- ❏ Disease Prevention
- ❏ Expected Body Image Changes
- ❏ Family Planning
- ☑ Family Systems
- ❏ Growth and Development
- ❏ Health and Wellness
- ❏ Health Promotion Programs
- ❏ Health Screening
- ☑ High Risk Behaviors
- ❏ Human Sexuality
- ❏ Immunizations
- ❏ Lifestyle Choices
- ☑ Principles of Teaching/Learning
- ❏ Self-Care
- ❏ Techniques of Physical Assessment

Psychosocial Integrity
- ❏ Abuse/Neglect
- ❏ Behavioral Interventions
- ❏ Chemical and Other Dependencies
- ❏ Coping Mechanisms
- ❏ Crisis Intervention
- ❏ Cultural Diversity
- ❏ End of Life Care
- ❏ Family Dynamics
- ❏ Grief and Loss
- ❏ Mental Health Concepts
- ❏ Psychopathology
- ❏ Religious and Spiritual Influences on Health
- ❏ Sensory/Perceptual Alterations
- ❏ Situational Role Changes
- ❏ Stress Management
- ☑ Support Systems
- ☑ Therapeutic Communications
- ❏ Therapeutic Environment
- ❏ Unexpected Body Image Changes

2007 NCLEX-RN® Test Plan Categories and Subcategories (Con.t)
Choose all areas included in the simulation

Physiologic Integrity
Basic Care and Comfort
- ☐ Assistive Devices
- ☑ Complementary and Alternative Therapies
- ☐ Elimination
- ☑ Mobility/Immobility
- ☑ Non-Pharmacological Comfort Interventions
- ☑ Nutrition and Oral Hydration
- ☐ Palliative/Comfort Care
- ☐ Personal Hygiene
- ☐ Rest and Sleep

Pharmacological and Parenteral Therapies
- ☐ Adverse Effects/Contraindications
- ☐ Blood and Blood Products
- ☐ Central Venous Access Devices
- ☑ Dosage Calculation
- ☐ Expected Effects/Outcomes
- ☑ Medication Administration
- ☑ Parenteral/Intravenous Therapies
- ☑ Pharmacological Agents/Actions
- ☐ Pharmacological Interactions
- ☐ Pharmacological Pain Management
- ☐ Total Parenteral Nutrition

Reduction of Risk Potential
- ☐ Diagnostic Tests
- ☑ Lab Values
- ☐ Monitoring Conscious Sedation
- ☐ Potential for Alterations in Body Systems
- ☐ Potential for Complications of Diagnostic Tests/Treatments/Procedures
- ☑ Potential for Complications from
- ☐ Surgical Procedures and Health
- ☐ Alterations
- ☐ System Specific Assessments
- ☑ Therapeutic Procedures
- ☑ Vital Signs

Physiologic Adaptation
- ☐ Alterations in Body Systems
- ☐ Fluid and Electrolyte Imbalances
- ☐ Hemodynamics
- ☐ Illness Management
- ☐ Infectious Diseases
- ☐ Medical Emergencies
- ☑ Pathophysiology
- ☐ Radiation Therapy
- ☑ Unexpected Response to Therapies

Scenario Progression Outline

Timing (Approximate)	Mannequin Actions	Expected Interventions	May Use the Following Cues
First 5 minutes	Temp 38.2 (tympanic) BP 118/74 P 100 reg strong RR 20 SpO2 90% Crackles bilaterally Hypoactive bowel sounds Moaning (slumped down in bed, sheets are twisted)	Wash hands Introduce self Acknowledge wife at bedside Check ID band and ask patient name, identify where he is and why	Role member providing cue: Cue:
Next 5-10 minutes	Vocal: "My name is Vernon Watkins and I had surgery on my stomach, this is my wife Martha" "I'm OK but my stomach is sore and I'm hungry" "It's sore so I guess it is about a 4-5"	Assess vital signs Conduct pain assessment Reposition patient and provide comfort measures Perform a shift assessment to include auscultation of lungs and pulse oximeter check Encourage deep breathing and coughing, use of incentive spirometer Review orders for diet, assess bowel sounds to determine bowel function, assess abdominal dressing.	Role member providing cue: Wife Cue: "Why does he still have pain, shouldn't you give him some more pain medication?" Wife: "Vernon is hungry, maybe if you give him something to eat, he'll feel better. He always likes Oatmeal with brown sugar and raisins when he doesn't feel well"
Final 15-20 minutes	P 112 B/P 134/88 RR 24 with loud crackles No bowel sounds Coughing (in regards to the incentive spirometer) "What is that?" "Can I have something to eat now?"	Recognize coughing, vital sign changes, and crackles indicate need for respiratory management (incentive spirometer use and cough and deep breathing). Provide patient and family teaching on use of incentive spirometer and splinting incision to deep breath and cough. Recognize that lack of bowel sounds indicate NOT to advance diet, need to report findings.	Role member providing cue: Wife Cue: "What is his blood pressure and pulse?" Wife: (in regard to incentive spirometer use) "He does not need that, it makes his stomach hurt more"

Debriefing / Guided Reflection Questions for this Simulation
(Remember to identify important concepts or curricular threads that are specific to your program)

1. How did you feel throughout the simulation experience?

2. Describe the objectives you were able to achieve?

3. Which ones were you unable to achieve (if any)?

4. Did you have the knowledge and skills to meet objectives?

5. Were you satisfied with your ability to work through the simulation?

6. To Observer: Could the nurses have handled any aspects of the simulation differently?

7. If you were able to do this again, how could you have handled the situation differently?

8. What did the group do well?

9. What did the team feel was the primary nursing diagnosis?

10. What were the key assessments and interventions?

11. Is there anything else you would like to discuss?

Complexity – Simple to Complex
Suggestions for changing the complexity of this scenario to adapt to different levels of learners:
- Patient could develop more serious postoperative complications such as a deep vein thrombosis or pulmonary embolism.
- Family dynamic issues that would be challenging, such as wife has early onset Alzheimers disease and has been taken care of by her husband at home.
- Patient could be verbally abusive and demanding of wife as well as to the nurses providing care.
- Patient could develop postop dementia.

CHAPTER 5

PRACTICAL SUGGESTIONS FOR IMPLEMENTING SIMULATIONS

Melissa Horn, MSN, RN, CFNP, CNN, CCTC, & Nina Carter, MEd, RN

*"...no industry in which human lives depend on
the skilled performance of responsible operators
has waited for unequivocal proof of the benefits
of simulation before embracing it...
Neither should anesthesiology."*

David M. Gaba, M.D.

Since the groundbreaking work on the integration of high-fidelity simulation into an anesthesia curriculum (Gaba, 1992), policy makers have taken note of the importance of technology in patient safety initiatives as well as in educating health professionals (Jha, Dunkin, & Bates, 2001). The information presented in previous chapters illustrates the various forces outside the walls of nursing academe that are influencing the movement toward use of instructional strategies with integrated technologies. Whether because of practice challenges imposed by health care delivery systems (Oermann & Garvin, 2002), nationwide initiatives toward improved health care safety and quality (IOM, 2004), or burgeoning societal demands on a workforce that is in short supply (National Sample Survey of Registered Nurses, 2005), nurse educators — like their clinical counterparts — find it necessary to strive for and maintain a state-of-the-art practice. With the challenges inherent in the health care environment and projections of future trends in the nursing workforce (Kowalski, 2001), preparing nursing professionals to meet these challenges is no trivial task. Simulation — a strategy that is gaining favor among nurse educators — is beginning to take its place as a learning modality in nursing curricula. Often, maintaining a state-of-the-art practice in which to educate tomorrow's nurses requires facing challenges created by scarce resources. However, with passion and some planning, nurse educators can overcome these challenges, and simulation can play a major role in doing so.

When simulation is incorporated into the education design, it can be used for introducing new concepts or skills and may produce enhanced learning outcomes. This is especially true for technical fields that require both a high level of critical thinking as well as psychomotor skills (Rauen, 2001). In a nursing assessment course, for example, students who participate in a simulation learn the principles of conducting an assessment, how to prioritize assessment data, and how to formulate a plan of care based on those data. Such an experience helps students gain confidence in assessment and decision making. If different student groups worked with various simulations, the learning from all groups could be shared to expand student experience (Engum, Jeffries, & Fisher, 2003; Jeffries, Woolf, & Linde, 2003).

Simulation requires the application of creativity while using some form of technology (Seropian, Brown, Gavilanes, & Driggers, 2004). Arguably, creativity is generally not a barrier for nursing faculty, but unfamiliar technology or the unwillingness to change traditional teacher-centered methods can pose a challenge to implementing simulation-based learning activities. However, the documented value of simulation as a teaching tool (Jeffries, 2005) should encourage more faculty to include this exciting option in their repertoire of teaching strategies. Unfortunately, a literature search in the "how-to" area of implementing simulation will yield some gaps, as was discovered during the NLN/Laerdal Simulation Study (see Appendix A). Therefore, based on experiences during the three-year NLN/Laerdal Simulation Study, this chapter is dedicated to the operational perspective of implementing a simulation, as well as lessons learned. In addition, since nurse educators have used low- and moderate-fidelity simulations for quite some time, this chapter focuses greater attention on implementing high-fidelity simulations.

The actual execution of a well-prepared simulation exercise is the culmination of careful planning, attention to detail, and collaborative efforts of faculty and administration. It is not unlike directing a theatrical production. There needs to be an appropriate venue, a simulation design, a detailed script, clear directions and expectations, actors, props, rehearsals, technical support, feedback, evaluation, and expert time management. This means investing greater effort than that expended for traditional teacher-centered instructional activities (Rauen).

Using simulation as a learner-centered strategy is not an impossible task, but it does benefit from some passion and a definite commitment. Why put in the extra effort, especially when empirical evidence of improved learning outcomes is in its early stages? Looking to simulated exercises utilized for public safety helps provide a rationale. For example, the Federal Aviation Administration requires full-scale emergency drills — high-fidelity simulations — in order to certify airports. These mock disasters require up to a year of planning and coordination with all public and emergency medical system stakeholders. They employ a well-planned scenario, live actors, and realistic simulated injuries, and they take place in an actual airport with the surrounding city, first responders, and local hospitals as the backdrop. The scenario and responses by personnel to the scenario are foundationally based on the local aviation emergency plan and operational requirements (Airport Security Rules for the Federal Aviation Administration, 2004). Although definitive empirical evidence may not be available regarding the value of simulation related to public safety, public administrators recognize the value of exercises that require active participation and application of theoretical knowledge and psychomotor skills, as well as decision making, communication, teamwork, and critical thinking.

Situations like these sound a great deal like nursing! Therefore, it is imperative that nurse educators explore these new technologies, incorporate simulations into their teaching repertoire, communicate their findings, and contribute to the evolving body of evidence about using simulation.

COMPONENTS FOR IMPLEMENTING SIMULATIONS

The following is an examination of various components used in high-fidelity simulations, along with some practical suggestions for implementation of simulation.

Venue

The first and foremost necessity is availability of a venue in which to conduct simulated learning activities. When space is at a premium, it can be difficult to engineer a high-fidelity simulation design. The next crucial element within the venue is the simulation equipment. Any simulation design is founded in the type of simulation equipment that is available for use. Finally, adequate access to the venue will dictate design and implementation of a simulation.

Design

A well-designed simulation incorporates educational best practices and simulation design criteria as described by Jeffries. Previous chapters provide in-depth information on these important elements.

Directions/Expectations

The course syllabus or simulation materials must contain specific, measurable objectives that correlate with stated curriculum outcomes. These need to be reviewed with the participants prior to engaging in the simulation. Participants also need clearly defined expectations as to their required performance and demonstration of knowledge and skills. It is also helpful to set boundaries with regard to expected behaviors related to interpersonal interactions, general safety, and specified roles within the scenario.

Script

A detailed script of the simulation provides clear information to participants regarding the location, time, setting, background history, individual players, available equipment, required performance, and theoretical knowledge and psychomotor skills required. The script should delineate the different roles in which students are expected to engage. Role descriptions need enough detail to assist the student in assuming the role. The script also serves as a guide to faculty involved in implementing the simulation.

"Actors"

In addition to student participants "acting" in the scenario, it is possible to use other faculty or volunteers to assume the role of patient, family member, or other health care personnel.

Props

For high-fidelity simulations, it is important to strive to recreate the environment depicted in the scenario by using realistic medical equipment, clothing, furnishings, lighting, and sounds.

Rehearsals

Faculty should rehearse a new simulation scenario and work out any "bugs" that might become apparent once implemented. Rehearsing also helps in setting a realistic timeline for the scenario.

Technical Support

High-fidelity simulations often use computerized human patient simulators or computer-based programs that require operators' knowledge of basic functions and troubleshooting. When using a human patient simulator, it often is helpful to the facilitator if an additional person operates the simulator while the facilitator directs the simulation, interacts with participants, and observes performance. It is possible, however, for the facilitator to accomplish both, if he/she is comfortable with the technology and supported by a videotaped record.

Feedback

Participants in a simulation require information from which decision making, behavior modification, and learning can take place. How, when, and what type of feedback is provided must be built into the simulation design as reflected in the script, along with consistent application among facilitators in all implementations.

Evaluation

The simulation design, user satisfaction, presence of educational practices, and learning outcomes are areas that should be evaluated in order to maintain integrity of the design and improve delivery of education.

Time Management

The well-designed simulation incorporates pre-scenario preparation, run-time of the scenario, and post-scenario reflection activities. Based on rehearsal-derived timelines, course design, facility restraints and support structures, keeping a simulation activity within the designated time allotment rests with the facilitator.

THE OPERATIONAL PLAN

From an operational perspective, there are phases to implementing a simulation that can be broken down into parts, similar to a project plan. Assuming that simulation space and equipment are available, the first phase requires development of the simulation scenario. In the next phase, providing staff development for colleagues new to the simulation design is critical, as is orienting participating students. Executing the simulation scenario comprises the third phase. Finally, evaluation takes place and revisions are made as necessary. Since other chapters provide in-depth information on simulation planning, development, and evaluation, only brief reference is made to these areas here, and detail is reserved for phase three (executing the simulation scenario).

Phase One: Scripting the Simulation

Once desired simulation equipment and appropriate facilities are in place, one can turn toward the goal of incorporating a high-fidelity simulation into a lesson plan. Often, preexisting case studies can be used to develop the simulation scenario. Instead of a desktop exercise, the case study needs to be brought to "life." As with all well-planned lessons, the implementation of a simulation design requires clear, attainable goals and objectives. The curriculum, curriculum map, and resulting course syllabus drive these goals and objectives. By using available curriculum documentation, faculty can decide on the complexity of simulations and methods for evaluating successful completion of objectives. Objectives may be the most important factor guiding the design, implementation, reflection, and evaluation of the simulation. When writing objectives, use of a taxonomy (for example, Bloom, 1984) supports correlation with the desired complexity of the simulation and fosters consistency with desired learning outcomes. For example, students in their first clinical/lab course would be overwhelmed by a very complex simulation that requires extensive critical thinking and rapid decision making. However, they could be quite successful with a simulation that involves a limited number of variables and requires minimal analysis.

It is important to remember that more "high-tech" equipment used in a simulation does not equate with a higher level of complexity. Likewise, a simulation that involves few or no technologies, such as interviewing a standardized patient, can be quite complex. The complexity of the simulation should increase as students' knowledge level expands, as they are expected to integrate more variables into their clinical decision making, and as they practice in increasingly ambiguous clinical simulations (Seropian et al.). At a novice level of complexity, faculty may conduct a focused simulation that requires students to assess lung sounds only. At an intermediate level of complexity, students may be asked to perform a comprehensive nursing assessment and record normal and abnormal findings. At higher levels of complexity, students may be required to formulate a nursing diagnosis or plan of care for a dyspneic patient as depicted by a human patient simulator. The latter scenario requires accurate data gathering and assessment; synthesis of various physical, psycho-social, and supporting history data; as well as defining the problem and designing care to resolve or manage it.

In addition to the design criteria discussed in previous chapters, the simulation also must accommodate logistic criteria such as time constraints, availability of space, support resources, class schedules, and number of students participating. Time for post-simulation reflection (debriefing) and a separate space for this portion of the simulation activity also must be considered. To ensure that the simulation meets all logistical requirements and maintains consistency during each implementation, faculty may find it helpful to use some written tools geared for two separate audiences. For colleagues involved in simulation activities, a written lesson plan or a simulation guide are good organizational tools and should contain information on setting up and running the simulation. For students who will be participating in the simulation activity, the syllabus or related course material should contain enough detail to help them understand how the simulation will be used in their learning activities and course objectives. It is helpful if the descriptive language in the simulation is consistent with correlating theoretical content, nursing diagnoses, and stated objectives.

Phase Two: Staff Development and Student Orientation

When implementing a student-centered simulation design that uses complex technology, it is imperative to provide participating faculty information on basic equipment operation, the role of technical support staff (if available), the simulation script itself, and any other resources. It also is important to provide background information on the simulation design, supporting data for using the design, and the logistics for implementing the simulation. If technical support staff are not available, it may be helpful to call upon technical support staff from the simulation equipment manufacturer as well as from faculty colleagues who have been trained as "super-users." It is important that faculty have resources and support to facilitate their comfort with the technology. Consider demonstrating the simulation by having faculty participate in role-play to support their insight on how students will experience the simulation as well as to define the role of faculty as facilitator. Opportunity for this type of staff development activity should be scheduled prior to the start of the term and repeated regularly to accommodate any new faculty.

Students' orientation should include content related to the simulation environment, expected conduct, safety rules, and resources. They should be provided with information on how they will use the syllabus, lab manual, or handouts in completing required assignments and activities. Specific to the simulation scenario, consider developing a matrix or table that describes the events taking place in the scenario, supporting data, possible actions, and required time frames for the expected actions. Define the different roles that students might be assigned and provide ample description of each in order to facilitate performance in each role. Students also must receive an orientation to the objectives of the simulation, expectations for pre-simulation content knowledge, expectations for participation and executing assigned roles, the purpose of post-simulation reflection (debriefing), and an orientation to any equipment to be used, its location, and expectations regarding its use. Students need to know if they will be expected to wear props or costumes to establish their roles, and they should be allowed to practice the simulation since the first experience with a high-fidelity simulator might distract from the objectives of the lesson.

Phase Three: Executing the Simulation Scenario

As noted in the preceding chapters, implementation should be consistent with the integrity of a well-designed simulation by including the following: objectives, fidelity, problem solving, student support, and reflective thinking (debriefing). In addition, educational practices of active learning, feedback, diverse learning styles, student/faculty interactions, time on task, collaboration, and high expectations should be considered when designing and implementing a simulation.

Pre-simulation setup.

Prior to the simulation session, the mannequin's physiologic responses based on the scripted scenario and anticipated student interventions will need to be programmed. The "stage" needs to be set using appropriate props; mannequins, with medical devices as called for in the scenario, need to be positioned; and all "costumes" and required equipment for students to complete the simulation must be on hand.

Pre-simulation student preparation.

A short time, for example ten minutes, may be spent to brief the students on the activity, review the objectives, and assign roles. If a pretest or preparatory questions are assigned prior to the simulation, validation of completion can be done at this time. It also is helpful to answer student questions regarding roles and expectations. Depending on the simulation, group size needs to be optimized to facilitate student participation and attainment of learning objectives. For example, scenarios requiring team interaction are more effective with fewer than six student participants.

Facilitating the simulation.

Have students step into their roles by obtaining props or costumes and setting the scene for them. This can be done by having them listen to a taped report or by verbally describing existing events as scripted in the scenario. Observe students as they role-play and interact with the mannequin, and provide additional data (that which cannot be simulated) if students request it. Rather than preventing students from making mistakes, allow the resulting physiologic responses of the mannequin to guide their thinking and interventions. Take care, however, not to progress to a catastrophic outcome. Unless the simulation objectives specifically call for it, such as a death and dying scenario, the scenario should end with a viable patient. Faculty also should refrain from having the very last scenario of the term depict poor patient outcomes. After simulation completion, students should remove costumes, step out of their roles, and relocate to an area outside the simulation staging site to engage in reflection. Scenario run time depends on the script; however, twenty minutes for the simulation and another twenty minutes for reflection worked well for participants in the NLN/ Laerdal Simulation Study (see Appendix A).

Phase Four: Evaluation

Student satisfaction data related to the simulation experience can be collected in the same manner that course evaluations are collected. It also is helpful to evaluate the presence of critical design and educational practice components by using survey instruments designed for this purpose, such as those mentioned in Appendix A. Based on these evaluation results and the learning outcomes achieved by students, the simulation should be modified to improve implementation and meet student learning needs.

Faculty might consider videotaping the simulation and/or reflective activity (Chau, Chang, Lee, Ip, Lee, & Wootten, 2001). They also might consider using simulation as a testing method, although further study in this area is warranted.

SAMPLE CASE IMPLEMENTATION

As part of the NLN/Laerdal Simulation Study (Appendix A), one associate degree nursing program elected to implement a simulation in the fourth semester Medical-Surgical II course. The program was equipped with a nursing lab facility and a SimMan® simulator. The required lab component consisted of one ninety-minute session per week in addition to theory and clinical components. Simulations using the human patient simulator were designed for eight different topics addressed in the course. The simulation related to care of the patient experiencing various types of shock is described here as an example of how to implement a simulation.

Phase One: Scripting the Simulation

During the summer semester, the nursing lab director and course coordinator collaborated to select one of the case studies currently used in the Medical-Surgical II course to develop into a simulation. This development took into account the available lab time, availability of simulation equipment, and access to a post-conference area. It required developing all simulation roles, based on number of participants, and outlining alternate plans (e.g., omitting a less critical or observational role or role supplementation by participating faculty in the event of a student absence). Descriptions of the simulation, student roles, expected participation, expected skill attainment, learning objectives, and evaluation methods were written into the course syllabus. Specific simulation tools were designed to provide students with background information on the case presentation, events occurring within the simulation, expected behaviors, and guiding questions. When writing the syllabus, particular care was taken to maintain consistent language with stated curriculum outcomes, learning objectives, and descriptions within the simulation. From these documents, the simulation was developed using the template provided in Figure 4-1. Instructions on facilitating the simulation, time frames, and required equipment were outlined, and resources were listed.

Phase Two: Staff Development and Student Orientation

Once the course materials were completed, it was necessary to help faculty learn about the new design and how to implement it. This was accomplished by creating a training video and a PowerPoint® presentation. A digital video camera was used to facilitate editing, image management, and content storage. Faculty volunteers, support staff, and a second-semester student participated in the making of the video. The video provided an example of how the simulation would be implemented, including pre-simulation preparation; explanation to participants regarding roles of students, technical support individuals, and faculty facilitators; and a reflection period. The last simulation of the term was chosen as the one that would be depicted in the video. Video participants were given an orientation to the human patient simulator and all equipment they would be expected to use. Faculty and all participants involved in the video rehearsed the simulation scenario prior to taping. The simulation featured a taped report, pages announced through a speaker system, and intravenous pump alarms to simulate a medical unit setting, in addition to the usual hospital equipment found in a nursing lab. Faculty indicated that even with their clinical knowledge and the simulation tool that described expected behaviors, they needed practice in order to execute the scenario expertly (Carter, 2004).

The materials were presented to all nursing faculty during faculty development week, prior to the start of the term. Faculty members who did not have simulation activities incorporated into their courses expressed a desire to develop them in the future. In addition, faculty who would be involved in the simulations received an orientation on the simulator, simulator computer application, and course design.

The same video was used for student orientation on the first day of lab. Students also received an orientation to the features of the simulator and the different roles they would be assigned. All students rotated through the different roles so that all got an opportunity to experience each one. The orientation included program materials, equipment, safety, expected participatory behaviors, interpersonal boundaries, theoretical preparation, and skills validation. Students were then allowed to participate in a practice simulation.

Phase Three: Executing the Simulation Scenario

Prior to class time, the simulator, video equipment, and required props were prepared. Details based on the scenario were manifest in coloring the simulator's lips and fingernails with blue-gray powdered eye shadow to simulate cyanosis or placing red dots on the body to simulate urticaria. Consistent with the scenario, observational data that could not be easily simulated were written on a small notepaper and taped to the affected body part such as "pulses absent" at the dorsalis pedis and post tibialis sites. The simulator was preprogrammed for the particular simulation and was tested prior to class time.

Class started promptly to facilitate completion of all required objectives. Each simulation was designed with two parts to facilitate student participation. Students were required to prepare for the simulation by completing pretest questions. As a group, the students reviewed questions, and further student inquiries were answered to provide clarification. Learning objectives also were reviewed. As was the practice at this school, skills validation for the simulation was accomplished the week prior to the simulation so that students could fully participate. Students were divided into two groups of four. They received role assignments and got into simple costumes set aside for the roles. During the first part of the simulation, two students participated and two were assigned to observe. These roles were reversed during part two of the simulation. This pre-simulation preparation time required a total of approximately ten minutes.

The simulation was started and progressed through to completion with a technical person assigned to control the simulator and video equipment and another faculty member acting as facilitator. Faculty were careful not to interrupt students and therefore to allow mistakes. Students were allowed to collaborate as a team to solve problems. Objective data were provided based on responses to patient presentation. Students had the opportunity to use actual medical equipment, call a physician, page a health care professional, or do anything else that would reasonably be accomplished in the hospital setting. The simulation scenarios were designed to run twenty minutes for each of the two parts with a ten-minute simulator reset time in between. During this time, students who participated in part one gave a nursing report to the next group. Then part two commenced. At the end of the simulation scenario, all students removed their "costumes" and relocated to an adjacent room to participate in the reflection period. Thirty minutes was set aside for the reflection (debriefing) time. A standard set of questions was reviewed, and there was open discussion and time to reflect quietly. Students wrote their impression of the simulation on a journaling form.

Phase Four: Evaluation

Students indicated that it took approximately two simulations (including the practice session) before they were confident enough to focus on the objectives and were less anxious about the activity (Carter). Sample comments on evaluations received at the end of the course included the following: "I finally understand what I'm supposed to be doing when I'm at clinical!" and "It's important that we have our simulation before our lecture exams because it helps to better understand the material," and "This was the best lab class I've had in the entire program." One student among the 62 participants did not feel that the simulation lab fit her preferred learning style because of the interactive group design but noted that it forced her to develop these skills. Students also indicated that they preferred not to have sessions videotaped, as this was a source of anxiety.

SUMMARY

The actual execution of a well-prepared simulation exercise is the culmination of careful planning, attention to detail, and collaborative efforts of faculty and administration. Information and practical guidelines to foster integration of high-fidelity simulation into courses have been provided throughout the chapter, as have discussions about the three phases of implementing simulations into the teaching environment: developing a scenario, providing for staff development, and executing the simulation. The operational aspects of implementing and executing a simulation scenario with references made to critical simulation design and educational practice requirements are all important elements to consider when incorporating a simulation experience into the teaching-learning experience. The sample case simulation, outlining each step of the implementation phase, provided in this chapter illustrates how using simulation in the teaching-learning environment provides for student-centered learning, provided it is well planned, carefully orchestrated, and rehearsed in advanced.

References

Airport Security Rules for the Federal Aviation Administration, 69 Fed. Reg. 6408 (Feb. 10, 2004) (to be codified at 14 C.F.R. pt.107).

Bloom, B. (1984) Taxonomy of educational objectives. White Plains, NY: Longman.

Carter, N. (2004, June). Nurse-SCAPES: Implementing simulated clinical and patient event staging. Presented at the 10th Biannual North American Learning Resource Centers Conference, Spokane, WA.

Chau, J., Chang, A., Lee, I., Ip, W., Lee, D., & Wootton, Y. (2001). Effects of using video-taped vignettes on enhancing students' critical thinking ability in a baccalaureate nursing programme. Journal of Advanced Nursing, 36(1), 112-119.

Engum, S. A., Jeffries, P. R., & Fisher, L. (2003). Intravenous catheter training system: Computer-based education versus traditional learning methods. American Journal of Surgery, 186(1), 67-74.

Gaba, D. M. (1992). Improving anesthesiologists' performance by simulating reality [editorial]. Anesthesiology, 76, 491-494.

IOM (Institute of Medicine). (2004). Keeping patients safe: Transforming the work environment of nurses. Washington, DC: National Academies Press.

Jeffries, P. R. (2005). A framework for designing, implementing and evaluating simulations used as teaching strategies in nursing. Nursing Education Perspectives, 26(2), 96-103.

Jeffries, P. R., Woolf, S., & Linde, B. (2003). Technology-based vs. traditional instruction: A comparison of two methods for teaching the skill of performing a 12-lead ECG. Nursing Education Perspectives, 24(2), 70-74.

Jha, A. K., Dunkin, B. W., & Bates, D. W. (2001). Simulator-based training and patient safety, making health care safer: A critical analysis of patient safety practices. (AHRQ Publication No. 01-E058). Rockville, MD: US Department of Health and Human Services.

Kowalski, K. (2001). Nursing work force of the future: The administrative perspective. Journal of Perinatal & Neonatal Nursing, 15(1), 8-15.

National Sample Survey of Registered Nurses, 2004, Preliminary findings. (2005). Rockville, MD: US Department of Health and Human Services, Health Resources Services Administration, Bureau of Health Professions. Available at http://bhpr.hrsa.gov/healthworkforce/reports/rnpopulation/preliminaryfindings.htm

Oermann, M. H., & Garvin, M. F. (2002). Stresses and challenges of new graduates in hospitals. Nurse Education Today, 22, 1-6.

Rauen, C. A. (2001). Using simulation to teach critical thinking skills. *Critical Care Nursing Clinics of North America, 13*(1), 93-103.

Seropian, M. A., Brown, K., Gavilanes, J. S., & Driggers, B. (2004). Simulation: Not just a manikin. *Journal of Nursing Education, 43*(4), 164-169.

CHAPTER 6
INTEGRATING GUIDED REFLECTION INTO SIMULATED LEARNING EXPERIENCES

Sharon Decker, MSN, RN, CCRN, CS

*"Teachers learn from their
students' discussions."*

Rashi

Health professions programs have been challenged (IOM, 2004) to use expanding technologies and support innovations throughout the educational process. These educational innovations include reforms in the methods, approaches, and settings used to provide clinical education, all in anticipation of the expectation that future "patient free" learning environments (such as simulation centers) will enhance the training of health professionals while minimizing harm to patients (Ziv, Small, & Wolpe, 2000).

Consistent with these recommendations to be more innovative in education practices, the National League for Nursing (2003) has challenged faculty to be creative and design new methods for clinical education in an effort to prepare graduates to thrive in the current health care environment. A question to consider is "Could integration of guided reflection into simulated learning experiences assist faculty in meeting this challenge?"

This chapter will present an overview of the concept of reflection, discuss the faculty's role in facilitating reflection, and provide a summary of the empirical findings to support the integration of guided reflection into learning experiences. Finally, this chapter will build on these data and present several frameworks to assist faculty in integrating guided reflection into simulated learning activities.

PHILOSOPHICAL UNDERPINNINGS AND DEFINITIONS OF REFLECTION

Dewey (1933) viewed reflection as an active, rigorous, and emotional initiative that promotes learning by building new knowledge on past experiences. According to Dewey, reflection is caused by "a state of doubt, hesitation, [or] perplexity" (p. 12) and requires the learner to be open-minded and willing to engage in the process. Dewey believed the learner needed to recognize the significance of an experience and stressed, "One can think reflectively only when one is willing to endure suspense and to undergo the trouble of searching" (p. 16).

Dewey divided the process of reflection into five phases: problem identification, collection of additional pertinent data, interpretation, hypothesis and reasoning, and testing or taking action. According to Dewey, problem identification could occur either during or after an experience and required both time and intellectualization. Once the problem has been identified, the learner collects additional relevant data and evaluates it for relevancy. During the third phase, interpretation, the individual seeks explanations and resources to broaden the understanding of the experience. As understanding and insight are achieved through a critical analysis of the experience, a hypothesis is formulated. This analysis leads to the final phase of testing, where the learner recognizes meaning and applies the acquired knowledge to new experiences.

Schön (1983), influenced by Dewey, describes two types of reflection: reflection-in-action and reflection-on-action. **Reflection-in-action** is the self-monitoring that occurs while an individual is engaged in an experience. This phase of reflection is stimulated by a puzzling or "interesting phenomenon with which the individual is trying to deal" (p. 50). Furthermore, Schön describes reflection-in-action as central to the "art" of practice. Reflection-in-action is the artistry displayed by the practitioner as knowledge from past experiences is integrated into an unfamiliar situation. By viewing new situations in the context of being "both similar to and different from the familiar one" (p. 138), the practitioner can make sense of uncertain situations and respond immediately. Schön (1987) states that the level of this response is influenced by the structure of the institution, the profession's body of knowledge, and the competence of the practitioners. **Reflection-on-action** (cognitive postmortem) is the conscious review of an interaction once it is completed. The goal of reflection-on-action is to critique an event in an effort to discover new understandings with the intent of applying the new knowledge to future practice (Schön, 1983).

Reflection is also a component of the cycle of experiential learning developed by Kolb (1984). The cycle of experiential learning provides a learning theory that integrates concrete (real-life) experiences, reflective observation (reflection or internalization of the experience), abstract conceptualization (looking for patterns and meanings), and active experimentation or building of new understandings. Kolb believes learning relies on reflective observations as an individual progresses from being involved to thinking about the experience and assimilating it into abstract concepts for future actions.

To summarize the reflective process as posed by Dewey, Schön, and Kolb, reflection is an active process of self-monitoring initiated by a state of doubt or puzzlement that occurs during or after an experience. As an essential component of experiential learning, reflection promotes insightfulness, which leads to the discovery of new knowledge with the intent of applying this knowledge to future situations. This view is reflected in the nursing literature by Kuiper and Pesut (2004), who suggest that reflective thinking is necessary for metacognitive skill acquisition and clinical reasoning or judgment, a perspective shared by Ruth-Sahd (2003), who proposes that the use of reflection decreases the gap between theory and practice.

According to some authorities, experience alone does not guarantee learning (Boud, Keogh, & Walker, 1985), but the integration of reflection promotes knowledge attainment from experience (Jarvis, 1992; Kuiper & Pesut; Wong, Kember, Chung & Yan, 1995). Yet we are cautioned by nurse authors (Tanner, 2006; Teekman, 2000) that learning from reflection is not automatic; it demands active involvement in a clinical experience (Teekman) and guidance throughout the reflective process (Johns, 1996; Tanner).

REFLECTION AND RELEVANCE TO NURSING

Benner, Hooper-Kyriakidis, and Stannard (1999) stress that learning does not occur without active participation nor is it guaranteed by the mere passage of time; it requires the learner to be open and engaged. In addition, these nurse experts state that development of clinical judgment requires the clinician to engage in "ongoing experiential learning, reflection, and dialogue with patients and their families" (p. 17). The importance of guided reflection is supported by Murphy (2004), whose research demonstrated that the instructional methodologies of articulation (oral and written) and focused reflection assisted the learner's application of theory to the clinical setting and promoted reasoning skills. Research conducted by Conway (1998) demonstrated that patient care varies according to the reflective abilities of the nurse. In this study, nurses who demonstrated minimal reflective abilities provided illness-oriented patient care, whereas nurses with reflective skills implemented care based on the individualized needs of the client. In addition, Paget (2001) identifies a perceived transferability of reflective practice to clinical practice when the concept of reflective practice is integrated into an academic curriculum. Participants in this study indicated that the changes in their clinical practice were influenced by the increased assertiveness and self-awareness achieved through the educational experience.

In summary, nurse experts have posed reflection as the art of nursing. The development of reflection as an art requires creativity and conscious self-evaluation over a period of time. But, once developed, reflection allows the clinician to deal with unique situations and could ultimately affect the administration of patient care. Therefore, nurse educators could hypothesize that if simulated learning experiences are based on the principles of experiential learning, and guided reflection is embedded into the simulated learning experience, then the experience should promote the insight needed for the development of clinical judgment that promotes quality patient care. This hypothesis needs to be studied systematically, but the assumptions are sound and should influence our teaching process.

CHARACTERISTICS OF A REFLECTIVE THINKER

Dewey stressed that an individual must have a willingness to participate in the reflective process. Westberg and Jason (2001) share this perspective and add the characteristic of being willing to learn. Other experts described "the skills" required to engage in the reflective process, including monitoring, analyzing, predicting, evaluating (Pesut & Herman, 1999), and the ability to take risks, be open, and have imagination (Westberg & Jason).

REFLECTIVE THINKING: INITIATING FACTORS, BARRIERS, AND OUTCOMES

Identified factors that initiate the reflective process include a perplexing event that causes feelings of doubt (Dewey) or puzzlement (Schön, 1983). Obstacles to engagement in reflection include the effects of previous education, socialization as a nurse, and an organizational culture that does not value the process (Glaze, 2002; Paget; Platzer, Blake, & Ashford, 2000).

Both negative and positive consequences of the reflective process have been identified in the literature, including a heightened perception of self-awareness (Henderson & Johnson, 2002), empathy (Gustafsson & Fagerberg, 2004), enhanced professional development, and building new knowledge upon existing knowledge and experience (Boud, 2001; Dewey; Schön, 1983). Some authorities suggest that clinicians who experience positive outcomes from the reflective process provide better patient care (Benner et al.; Pesut & Herman).

Pesut and Herman claim the quality of patient care provided by a nurse is directly related to the amount and depth of reflective thinking in which the individual engages. According to these authorities, reflective practitioners are not just interested in what worked, they are curious about what did not work in an effort to modify future actions to improve patient care. Benner et al. think that reflection sensitizes the learner to "context-sensitive patient responses" and the "meaning of specific responses" (p. 58), which promote the development of clinical judgment and thus enhance patient care.

Negative outcomes identified were feelings of personal distress, self-doubt, isolation, and insecurity (Boud; Haddock, 1997; Kotzabassaki, Panou, Domou, Karabagli, Koursopoulou, & Ikonomou, 1997). Boud (2001) and Johns (1996) indicate that the reflective process does not automatically promote learning and the development of insight. Boud cautions that the reflective process "can become diffuse and disparate so that conclusions or outcomes may not emerge" (p. 3), and without appropriate guidance the desired outcomes of the reflective process may not be achieved (Boud et al.). Furthermore, the outcomes of the reflective process are influenced by the effectiveness of the facilitator (Paget).

Johns (2004) also stresses that because reflection can produce negative thoughts, a guide needs to support the learner throughout the process. The role of the guide, according to Johns, is to help the learner "think about things differently" (p. 77); to "infuse the practitioner with courage to take action to resolve contradictions" (p. 79); and to "...listen to the practitioner's story, ...and support the practitioner to face up to anxiety rather than defend against it...to see beyond themselves, to reveal possibilities for responding in new, more effective ways within similar situations,...to nurture commitment and responsibility, [and] to challenge and support practitioners to act on new insights" (p. 74). To foster this experience, the guide needs to accept the relevance of the process and create a safe environment in which the expression of feelings and group interactions are supported and remain confidential (Ruth-Sahd). Table 6-1 presents features of a safe environment for guided reflection, while Table 6-2 summarizes the key responsibilities of the facilitator during guided reflection.

Table 6-1. Facilitator's Guide for Establishing a Safe Environment for Reflection
1. Plan the experience as a learning opportunity
2. Select or develop a tool to facilitate an open discussion
3. Secure a private, comfortable environment
4. Arrange seating in a circular design
5. Limit participants to those directly involved in the simulated learning experience (3 to 5 students)
6. Allow time for reflection (20 to 30 minutes)
7. Introduce the session; emphasize the objectives and the importance of confidentiality and trust
8. Allow for a circular movement between and among the questions used to facilitate the discussion

Table 6-2. Facilitator's Responsibilities during Guided Reflection
1. Be supportive
2. Establish and uphold ground rules related to confidentiality and trust
3. Create an environment based on trust
4. Encourage and engage group members in dialogue
5. Listen attentively
6. Help the learner deal with feelings of ambiguity
7. Monitor and facilitate group dynamics
8. Promote the recognition of patterns
9. Facilitate the development of insight
10. Facilitate the transfer of knowledge
11. Nurture commitment to action
12. Challenge the learner to initiate change
13. Support the learner to act on her/his insights

(Carkhuff, 1996; Johns, 2004; Westberg & Jason, 2001)

Westberg and Jason stress that the skills required to engage in the reflective process can be learned. But sufficient time and appropriate learning experiences (real or simulated) are needed to promote this process. The development of insight could be lost if the individual is not allowed time to explore and connect the new learning. Therefore, nurse educators are challenged to plan learning experiences that 1) initiate feelings of perplexity, 2) require the learner to build upon past knowledge and skills, 3) require active participation in a patient care situation, 4) demand the engagement of critical thinking, and 5) support reflection. The learning environment for these experiences needs to support a culture of trust and facilitate both reflection-in-action and reflection-on-action.

FACILITATING THE DEVELOPMENT OF REFLECTIVE THINKING

Various techniques are posed to promote the development of clinical judgment through reflection. These methods vary from individual methods, such as inquiry journals, to structured group experiences. Strategies identified to support individual reflection include journal writing (Paget; Riley-Doucet & Wilson, 1997), audiotaped journaling (Kuiper, 2005), and email-based dialogues (Henderson & Johnson). The use of these strategies has been shown to enhance the learner's feelings of self-awareness and self-confidence. Structured group experiences provide learners with different perspectives and assist students in acquiring the skill of providing constructive critiques (Carkhuff, 1996; Westberg & Jason).

Schön (1987) proposes the use of a reflective practicum to enhance the process of reflection. A reflective practicum is a realistic event strategically planned by faculty to promote professional artistry. The environment for this learning event is described as being similar to those created in studios. Schön feels this unique environment allows "freedom to learn by doing in a setting relatively low in risk, with access to coaches who initiate students into the 'traditions of the calling' and help them, by 'the right kind of telling,' to see on their own behalf and in their own way what they need most to see" (p. 17). This reflective practicum has considerable likeness to the learning environment and experience depicted by the simulation framework proposed by Jeffries (2005). The simulation framework discussed in chapter 3 emphasizes that for learning to be successful, the experience needs to be designed around the characteristics of objectives, fidelity, problem solving, cues and debriefing.

STRATEGIES TO GUIDE REFLECTION

Guided reflection can be integrated into the simulated experience to promote both reflection-in-action and reflection-on-action through the use of Socratic questioning. The principles of Socratic questioning allow for the complexity of questions to be elevated as students acquire knowledge and skills (Caputi & Engelmann, 2004). Questions need to be developed, written on prompt cards, and integrated strategically into each simulation based on the learning objectives and the abilities of the students. For example, to promote reflection-in-action for learners who are at the novice or advanced beginner stages (Benner, 1984), a faculty member could be visually present in the patient care setting to guide the student's thoughts and actions at designated intervals. Lower level questioning could be interjected, such as the following: "I noticed you elevated the head of the bed (very good); explain the rationale behind your action." Or, to guide the student to another action, the faculty member may ask, "Is there any other action you could initiate that would also help your patient's oxygenation status?"

A strategy combining the use of role modeling and thinking out loud could be used to demonstrate reflection-in-action across the spectrum of learning. Imagine students observing two faculty "thinking out loud" as they provide patient care. Faculty using this technique of reflection-in-action could role model critical thinking and reflective thinking as they demonstrate principles of prioritization, delegation, and communication. The complexity of the scenario would be designed and scripted to meet specific learning needs of the students. This learning experience should integrate a debriefing session to allow students time to recognize and reflect on their learning. Additional scenarios that require learners to provide patient care based on the same objectives could be developed and initiated by students immediately after the debriefing session to support the transfer of learning.

Numerous frameworks have been developed to assist faculty in the process of facilitating reflection-on-action. Johns (2004) describes the reflective cycle outlined by Gibbs in 1988, noting that it assists in the transfer of insight into practice through the use of questioning. Questions using the Gibbs' reflective cycle are posed, guiding the discussion by 1) beginning with a description of the event, "What happened?", 2) progressing to a discussion of feelings, "What were you thinking and feeling?", 3) evaluating the experience, "What was good and bad about the experience?", 4) engaging in analysis, "What sense can you make of the situation?", 5) performing a self-critique, "What else could you have done?", and 6) generating an action plan, "If it arose again, what would you do?" (p.17).

Johns (1995) developed a model for structured reflection that provided cue questions based on Carper's four ways of knowing (Carper, 1978) to support the process of guided reflection. Carper's fundamental patterns of knowing in nursing include four fundamental, interrelated ways of knowing. The identification of four patterns that allow for "an increased awareness of the complexity and diversity of nursing knowledge" (p. 21). The first way of knowing, empirical, is aimed at developing theoretical explanations. Empirical knowledge is knowledge that can be methodically organized into general laws and theories. The second way of knowing, aesthetics, can be traced to Dewey and is the difference between recognition and perception. The third way of knowing is personal knowledge and involves the relationships be-tween patients and the nurse. Personal knowledge, according to Carper, is the most essential in understanding what health means to the individual. Ethics, the final way of knowing, represents the moral component and consists of professional obligations, norms, and ethical codes.

Utilizing the framework provided by Johns (2004, p.18), the facilitator poses questions to stimulate thinking in each of Carper's four ways of knowing and to stimulate thoughtful reflection. Examples include the following

Empirical	"What knowledge informed or might have informed you?"
Aesthetic	"What particular issues seem significant to pay attention to?"
Personal	"What factors influenced the way you felt, thought or responded?"
Ethical	"To what extent did you act for the best and in tune with your values?
Reflection	"How might you respond more effectively given this situation again?"

A modification to the model for structured reflection was derived by this author from the outcome of a research study and input received from experts in grounded theory methodology. The Facilitator's Tool for Guided Reflection Sessions (see Table 6-3) was used in a pilot study that was part of the NLN/Laerdal Simulation Study (see Appendix A). The purpose of this pilot study was to explore how beginning nursing students prioritize patient care during a simulated learning experience using a high-fidelity mannequin. Findings revealed that students at the beginning level used trial and error decision making that demonstrated minimal knowledge transfer, and the patient care they planned was prioritized around the need to complete tasks (Decker, 2006).

Table 6-3. Facilitator's Tool for Guided Reflection Sessions	
Ways of Knowing	**Open ended Questions/Statements to Encourage Reflection-on-Action**
Empirical	• Talk to me about the knowledge, skills, and experiences you have that helped you provide patient care during this simulated experience.
Aesthetic	• Talk to me about the problem your patient was having. • What was your main goal during this simulation?
Personal	• Tell me what influenced your actions during the scenario. • Talk to me about how this experience made you feel. • Talk to me about how satisfied you are with the actions you initiated during this scenario.
Ethical	• Talk to me about how your personal values and beliefs influenced your actions during this experience.
Reflection	• Talk to me about how you knew what to do during this situation. • What would you do differently if we went back into the patient's room and repeated the scenario right now? • Discuss how you will use what was learned in this experience in the future?

(Johns, 1995)

Further research is needed to expand this exploration and provide the evidence to demonstrate the learning and patient care outcomes achieved when guided reflection is integrated into a simulated learning experience. This research could explore how the use of guided reflection in simulated learning experiences affects students' development of clinical judgment throughout a program. Other questions to be posed for the integration of reflection into simulated learning experiences, as outlined in Table 6-4, need to be investigated. These explorations could demonstrate nurse educators' commitment to evidence-based teaching as well as meeting the challenges of being more innovative and of integrating expanded technologies into the educational process.

Table 6-4. Research Question to Be Addressed when Integrating Reflection into Simulated Learning Experiences
1. What conditions promote reflection during a simulated learning experience?
2. What are the benefits and risks of integrating reflection into a simulated learning experience for both the learner and the educator?
3. Does the integration of reflection into a simulated learning experience affect learning outcomes?
4. Does the integration of reflection into a simulated learning experience promote the development of clinical judgment?
5. Is insight gained during reflection transferred to the patient care setting? If so, how does this affect patient care outcomes?
6. Do past learning experiences impact the outcome of an experience that integrates guided reflection?

SUMMARY

Kuiper and Pesut claim both critical thinking (cognitive) and reflective thinking (metacognitive) skills are needed for the development of clinical reasoning (judgment). Yet empirical evidence is still needed to validate this claim and demonstrate how clinical judgment can be promoted through the use of an innovative teaching strategy that uses guided reflection in a simulated learning experience. Nurse educators have been challenged to be innovators in the process of educational reform in an effort to promote student learning and acquisition of competence. The integration of guided reflection into simulated experiences could provide faculty with a unique strategy to meet this challenge while providing quality education. However, research is still needed to validate this claim and demonstrate best educational practices for facilitating the process.

REFERENCES

Benner, P. (1984). *From novice to expert: Excellence and power in clinical nursing practice*. Menlo Park, CA: Addison-Wesley.

Benner, P., Hooper-Kyriakidis, P., & Stannard, D., (1999). *Clinical wisdom and interventions in critical care: A thinking-in-action approach*. Philadelphia: W. B. Saunders.

Boud, D., Keogh, R., & Walker, D. (1985). Promoting reflection in learning: A model. In D. Boud, R., Keogh, & D. Walker (Eds.), *Reflection: Turning experience into learning* (pp. 18-40). London: Routledge.

Boud, D. (2001). Using journal writing to enhance reflective practice. *New Directions for Adult and Continuing Education, 90*, 9-17.

Caputi, L. & Engelmann, L. (2004). *Teaching nursing: The art and science* (Vol. 1). Glen Ellyn, IL: College of DuPage Press.

Carkhuff, M. H. (1996). Reflective learning: Work groups as learning groups. *Journal of Continuing Education in Nursing, 27*(5), 209-214.

Carper, B. A. (1978). Fundamental patterns of knowing in nursing. *Advances in Nursing Science, 1*, 13-23.

Conway, J. (1998). Evolution of the species "expert nurse." An examination of the practical knowledge held by expert nurses [Electronic version]. *Journal of Clinical Nursing, 7*(1), 75-82.

Decker, S. (2006, June). Simulation and the development of critical thinking: A qualitative exploration. Poster presented at the 11th Biennial North American Learning Resource Center Conference, Philadelphia, PA.

Dewey, J. (1933). *How we think: A restatement of the relation of reflective thinking to the educative process*. Lexington, KY: D. C. Heath.

Glaze, J. (2002). Stages in coming to terms with reflection: Student advanced nurse practitioners' perceptions of their reflective journeys. *Journal of Advanced Nursing, 37*(3), 265-272.

Gustafsson, C., & Fagerberg, I. (2004). Reflection, the way to professional development? *Journal of Clinical Nursing, 13*(3), 271-280.

Haddock, J. (1997). Reflection in groups: Contextual and theoretical considerations within nursing education and practice. *Nursing Education Today, 17*, 381-385.

Henderson, P., & Johnson, M. H. (2002). An innovative approach to developing the reflective skills of medical students [Electronic version]. *BMC Medical Education, 2*(4), 1-4.

IOM (Institute of Medicine). (2004). *Academic health centers: Leading change in the 21st century*. Washington, DC: National Academies Press.

Jarvis, P. (1992). Reflective practice and nursing. *Nurse Education Today, 12*, 174-181.

Jeffries, P. R. (2005). A framework for designing, implementing, and evaluating simulations used as teaching strategies in nursing. *Nursing Education Perspectives, 26*(2), 96-103.

Johns, C. (1995). Framing learning through reflection within Carper's fundamental ways of knowing in nursing. *Journal of Advanced Nursing, 22*(2), 226-234.

Johns, C. (1996). Visualizing and realizing caring in practice through guided reflection. *Journal of Advanced Nursing, 24*(6), 1135-1143.

Johns, C. (2004). *Becoming a reflective practitioner* (2nd ed.). Malden, MA: Blackwell.

Kolb, D. A. (1984). *Experiential learning: Experience as the source of learning and development.* Englewood Cliffs, NJ: Prentice-Hall.

Kotzabassaki, S., Panou, M., Domou, F., Karabagli, A., Koursopoulou, B., & Ikonomou, U. (1997). Nursing students' and faculty's perceptions of the characteristics of "best" and "worst" clinical teachers: A replication study. *Journal of Advanced Nursing, 26*, 817-824.

Kuiper, R. A. (2005). Self-regulated learning during a clinical preceptorship: The reflections of senior baccalaureate nursing students. *Nursing Education Perspectives, 26*(6), 351-356.

Kuiper, R. A., & Pesut, D. J. (2004). Promoting cognitive and metacognitive reflective reasoning skills in nursing practice: Self-regulated learning theory. *Journal of Advanced Nursing, 45*(4), 381-391.

Murphy, J. I. (2004). Using focused reflection and articulation to promote clinical reasoning: An evidence-based teaching strategy. *Nursing Education Perspectives, 25*(5), 226-231.

National League for Nursing. (2003). *Position statement: Innovation in nursing education: A call to reform*. [Electronic version.] Available: http://www.nln.org/aboutnln/PositionStatements/innovation.htm.

Paget, T. (2001). Reflective practice and clinical outcomes: Practitioners' views on how reflective practice has influenced their clinical practice. *Journal of Clinical Nursing, 10*(2), 204-214.

Pesut, D. J., & Herman, J. (1999). *Clinical reasoning: The art and science of critical and creative thinking*. Albany, NY: Delmar.

Platzer, H., Blake, D., & Ashford, D. (2000). Barriers to learning from reflection: A study of the use of group work with post-registration nurses. *Journal of Advanced Nursing, 31*(5), 1001-1008.

Riley-Doucet, C., & Wilson, S. (1997). A three-step method of self-reflection using reflective journal writing. *Journal of Advanced Nursing, 25*(5), 964-968.

Ruth-Sahd, L. A. (2003). Reflective practice: A critical analysis of data-based studies and implications for nursing education. *Journal of Nursing Education, 42*(11), 488-497.

Schön, D. A. (1983). *The reflective practitioner: How professionals think in action.* New York: Basic Books.

Schön, D. A. (1987). *Educating the reflective practitioner.* Hoboken, NJ: Jossey-Bass.

Tanner, C. A. (2006). Thinking like a nurse: A research-based model of clinical judgment in nursing. *Journal of Nursing Education, 45*(6), 204-211.

Teekman, B. (2000). Exploring reflective thinking in nursing practice. *Journal of Advanced Nursing, 31*(5), 1125-1135.

Westberg, J., & Jason, H. (2001). *Fostering reflection and providing feedback*. New York: Springer Publishing.

Wong, F. K. Y., Kember, D., Chung, L. Y. F., & Yan, L. (1995). Assessing the level of student reflection from reflective journals. *Journal of Advanced Nursing, 22*, 48-57.

Ziv, A., Small, S. D., & Wolpe, P. R. (2000). Patient safety and simulation-based medical education. *Medical Teacher, 22*(5), 489-495.

CHAPTER 7
EVALUATING SIMULATIONS
Pamela R. Jeffries, DNS, RN, FAAN, & Kristen J. Rogers, MSN, RN

"How to tell students what to look for

without telling them what to see

is the dilemma of teaching."

Lascelles Abercrombie

Evaluating teaching-learning strategies and new instructional activities such as the use of simulations in the nursing curriculum can be challenging, but it is important to do in order to ensure that outcomes are being achieved. When implementing learning activities, nurse educators face the challenge of selecting appropriate evaluation strategies. When the learning strategy is simulation, various formative and summative evaluation methods can be utilized. This chapter will present an overview of selected evaluation methods. Also included in the chapter is a review of several instruments educators can use to evaluate the effectiveness of the simulation design.

In choosing the appropriate evaluation strategies, the educator needs to determine whether the focus is on the learner's progress toward goal attainment (formative), or the learner's attainment of a goal (summative). In **formative evaluation**, learners are provided with feedback from the educator and also conduct self-reflection, which allow them the opportunity to improve their performance (Oermann & Gaberson, 2006). Particular formative strategies can include mid-term surveys, one-minute papers, concept maps, and anecdotal notes. In **summative evaluation**, which occurs at the end of a learning period, learners are provided with feedback about their attainment of the learning objectives. Summative evaluation strategies can include multiple-choice tests, skills performance tests, rating scales, and criterion-based concept maps. Whether the evaluation is formative or summative, however, it provides information about learners' progress, competencies, skills, or knowledge. Involving learners in the evaluation process helps them see how well the objectives of the course have been met, in addition to identifying their own strengths, areas for improvement, and competency level.

HOW TO EVALUATE THE USE OF SIMULATIONS

In general, evaluation depends on the educators' philosophy and beliefs about the concept, which will influence frequency and timing, methods, and how results are interpreted and used (Bourke & Ihrke, 2005). When simulations are used as a teaching-learning activity, evaluation can involve information about the instructional design of the simulation itself; the educational practices incorporated in the simulation to promote learning; timing; clarity of the simulation; and the overall flow and fidelity of the simulation. In addition, evaluation can be conducted at the end of a teaching-learning activity using simulations to verify and document specific learning outcomes the educator wants to measure, including teaching-learning effectiveness and specific competencies the simulation was designed to teach (e.g., care of a patient with chest tubes).

Evaluation using simulations involves a systematic process just like any other evaluation plan. These steps include: 1) identifying the purpose of the evaluation; 2) determining a time frame to evaluate; 3) identifying when to evaluate; 4) developing an evaluation plan;

5) selecting the evaluation instrument(s); 6) collecting data, and 7) interpreting the data (Billings & Halstead, 2005).

Identifying the Purpose of the Evaluation

In evaluation, one of the first steps is to design the evaluation questions that the data will answer since clarity of what is being evaluated is needed and important to conduct the evaluation. The questions can be focused, such as whether students can perform a selected skill set or care for a specific type of client, or they may be broad and encompassing, for example, whether there is a higher order of thinking involved when students are immersed in a teaching-learning environment using simulations. The purpose of the evaluation should be clear to students, faculty, and all involved.

Determining a Time Frame to Evaluate

The time frame for evaluation is partly determined by whether the evaluation is for formative or summative purposes. If it is for formative purposes, the evaluation serves as more of an assessment of performance, at a point before the end of the learning experience, and will most likely occur in the middle of the experience or after a critical event has taken place. Formative evaluation assesses students' progress or achievement of a specific goal by the end of an instructional unit or assesses a particular teaching-learning activity, instruction, or scenario. However, only selected parts of the teaching-learning activity are evaluated as opposed to the entire learning experience, course, or program.

Summative evaluation may include using a simulation to assess students' competence on selected critical behaviors, skills, and knowledge at the end of the course. The focus is on a whole event or concept area for which outcomes need to be measured. Measured outcomes may involve a grade or a pass/fail judgment, and they may entail remediation if this is a required competency students need before progressing on in the course or curriculum.

Identifying When to Evaluate

Determining when to evaluate also depends on whether the simulation evaluation is formative or summative. If formative, the evaluation occurs after the students have participated in the simulation activity, but while there is still time in the course for them to strengthen their weak areas and improve their performance if it did not meet expectations. If summative, most likely for a grade or to document a specific competency level before the learner can progress, the evaluation typically occurs at the end of the course or at the end of a module or component of instruction.

Developing an Evaluation Plan

When implementing simulations or any other type of innovative teaching strategy for students, an evaluation plan should be developed, as mentioned, to ensure students are indeed learning from the activity. The plan needs to include the specific type of evaluation, exactly how the evaluation will be conducted, who will do it, instruments or tools to be used, and the intended outcomes or activities to be evaluated. When several educators are involved in the course, evaluation planning needs to include all of them. As the last, and very important, component in the teaching-learning process, a well-organized evaluation can be implemented easily if all components have been defined and prepared before the evaluation actually occurs.

Selecting the Evaluation Instrument(s)

Once the educator identifies the variables to be assessed, the measurement instrument(s) can be selected. These depend on the evaluation framework. One instrument is the CIPP model (Stufflebeam & Webster, 1994), which specifies context, input, process, and product. Another possible instrument to use is a naturalistic, constructivist model (Lincoln & Guba, 1985), in which the values, concerns, and issues of those involved in the evaluation (students, faculty, clients, and administrators) are taken into account. Different evaluation models and instruments are described in the simulation literature (Morgan & Cleave-Hogg, 2000; Robertson, 2006; Weller, 2004; Winston & Szarek, 2005), depending on what product, outcome, or component is being measured. The instruments chosen should be reliable and valid measures of the component being assessed. Many instruments can be adapted to elicit information about a number of nursing activities. Commonly used types of simulation instruments are described below.

Questionnaires.

This instrument is a self-report method in which an individual responds to questions in writing on paper or a form. Items in the questionnaire need to be concise, clear, and simple, so the respondent can understand what is being asked (Polit & Hungler, 1995). Examples of instruments frequently used in simulations include measures of self-confidence about caring for a client in a clinical setting, presence of key simulation design features present in the simulation itself, and critical thinking. The measure of critical thinking has varied across studies, with researchers using different questionnaire instruments: Facione and Facione's (1996) California Critical Thinking Skills Tests (CCTST) (Chau, Chang, Lee, Ip, Lee, & Wootton, 2001), their California Critical Thinking Disposition Inventory (CCTDI) (Ravert, 2002), or an instructor-developed critical thinking inventory to assess students' critical thinking abilities. The researcher and the study purpose guide the choice of instrument to measure critical thinking. Winston and Szarek used questionnaires as the evaluation instrument to measure satisfaction with the experience, understanding of content, and knowledge application of 136 students in a problem-based learning program for an integrated curriculum involving a human patient simulator. In an obstetrical simulation using Noelle™ equipment, researchers used questionnaires to elicit students' perceptions of the clinical activity (Robertson).

Observation.

This type of evaluation involves an evaluator, typically an instructor or another trained participant, observing skills or critical behaviors of students while they participate in the simulation. Observation or a performance appraisal is useful for evaluating skill performance, skill competency, development of selected values and attitudes, and communication skills. Ideally, students will be provided feedback about what has been observed immediately after the simulated event in the debriefing or guided reflection period that follows the simulation itself. Informing students immediately after the behavior allows time for remediation and correction of any incorrect activity or skill. Examples of observation in simulation include observing communication skills, collaborative skills with members of an interdisciplinary team, and critiquing an advanced skill (e.g., airway management) that would be built into the simulation itself.

In various simulation studies using observation data (Aronson, Rosa, Anfinson, & Light, 1997; Cioffi, 2001; Johnson, Zerwic, & Theis, 1999; Peterson & Bechtel, 2000; Thiele, Holloway, Murphy, Pardavis, & Stuckey, 1991), researchers measured self-confidence and clinical judgments. One such study (Bramble, 1994) found that structured simulations encouraged students to think as opposed to memorize. Morgan and Cleave-Hogg evaluated medical students' performance using an anesthesia simulator, five independent evaluators, and standardized performance evaluation criteria. The correlation coefficient of interrater reliability was 0.87, suggesting that the simulator was a reliable assessment method to measure students' performance.

Checklists.

In nursing, checklists often are used to evaluate an expected student behavior. Often, checklists indicate that the behavior is met or not met. However, weighted checklists can be designed in which a scoring mechanism is included for each item, giving more important behaviors on the checklist more weight (e.g., 2 points instead of 1 point). This type of instrument is helpful for both formative and summative evaluation. Checklists are easy to complete and can be used for many purposes, such as assessing skill performance outcomes in the psychomotor realm. If the learning outcome relates to performance of a beginning skill (e.g., catheterization), the educator, using a checklist, clarifies for the learner the steps or the required performance criteria. Skill performance also can be videotaped, which provides learners an opportunity to assess their own performance (Billings & Halstead) and provides educators flexibility regarding when and where they give constructive feedback to learners. For example, the tape can be reviewed in the faculty member's office at a later time. Winters, Hauck, Riggs, Clawson, and Collins (2003) found that videotaping skill performance was positive for students and instructors alike; students report increased confidence when performing skills in the clinical setting after reviewing their videotaped performance along with the instructor, and faculty reported improvement in students' abilities to perform the videotaped skills in the clinical setting.

Attitude scales.

This type of instrument allows the educator to measure how the student feels about a particular subject at the moment the individual is tested. The measures typically have Likert scale responses from, for example, strongly agree to strongly disagree. Several types of attitude scales are used in simulation evaluation, such as measures of self-efficacy and satisfaction with the strategy as a method of instruction. Using a Likert scale format, Jeffries, Woolf, and Linde (2003) and Engum, Jeffries, and Fisher (2003) asked students to rate various aspects of an interactive simulated experience and a traditional learning experience.

Journal/diary.

Journaling is a type of self-reporting students can do that is a narrative of their reflections, activities, and feelings about the performance. Journals can be a one-time assignment or a continuous evaluation method throughout the course or clinical experience so the educator can track reflections and experiences across time. The value of the tool depends on how it is planned and constructed and how it is used (Bourke & Ihrke). Jenkins and Turick-Gibson (1999) used student journals to measure critical thinking when using simulations. Weller used thematic analysis of students' written comments when studying 33 fourth-year medical students to evaluate the use of simulation-based teaching in the context of management.

Anecdotal notes.

This type of student evaluation with simulation is also described in the literature (Hample, Herbold, Schneider, & Sheeley, 1999; Jenkins & Turick-Gibson; Peterson &

Bechtel). Anecdotal notes are the instructor's notations about the student's performance or behavior after an observed event (e.g., a simulation activity). Clear objectives should be identified for this measurement since its direct value is related to the objectives being evaluated. Anecdotal notes are more valuable when they are collected over time, summarized, and assessed for patterns and trends. A continuous assessment of the learner decreases one-time biases and reflects a more fair judgment of the student or event.

Collecting Data

Evaluation data will need to be collected after all the simulation steps are completed by students. The method selected determines how one will collect the data and the time needed to do the task. Various factors should be considered when collecting the data: data source, amount of data being collected, timing of the data collection, and whether the data collection is informal or formal. Informal data collecting includes spontaneous remarks from students that educators then use to draw conclusions about satisfaction with and learning from the event. In other cases, a formalized evaluation process takes place in which structured evaluation tools are used at a specific time. Timing of the data collection depends on the number of variables being assessed, and caution should be taken not to overburden students with data collection because results can be affected by this factor.

Interpreting the Data

In this step, the evaluation responses are interpreted to answer the evaluation questions that were asked before the process was implemented. Data must be put in a usable form so educators can understand their meaning and implications. Data interpretation should consider the context of the evaluation process, the frame of reference, objectivity, and legal and ethical issues (Billings & Halstead).

EVALUATING THE SIMULATION ACTIVITY ITSELF

Evaluation of the simulation itself should occur during three different phases: 1) design/development; 2) implementation, and 3) outcomes. Each phase will be described with example evaluation measures for each.

The Design/Development Phase

In order to evaluate the design and development of a simulation that is created by nurse educators, Jeffries, Childs, Decker, Horn, Hovancsek, Childress, Rogers, Feken, Spunt, & Politi, (2004) developed the Simulation Design Scale (SDS) (see Table 7-1). The purpose of this tool is to provide the educator with information/feedback that can be utilized to improve the simulation design and implementation. The SDS provides measures of the importance of each design feature of the simulation in addition to the degree each design feature is adequately embedded within the simulation design.

Table 7-1. Simulation Design Scale (SDS): Components	
Component	Description
Objectives/Information	Clear objectives and time frame for the simulation are needed by students before the simulation begins. Information needs to be provided on what learners need to know and what they are expected to learn.
Student Support	Student support is offered before, during, and after a simulation. Support includes providing information and direction to the student prior to the simulation. During the simulation, cues can be provided to the students participating in the simulation via a lab test, a CXR report, a phone call from a physician or a nurse manager, or in other ways. After a simulation, support is provided during the debriefing. Students find the debriefing part of the simulation a most important aspect; instructors are helpful when they correct misinformation or inappropriate actions that happened in the scenario, in addition to emphasizing components that should have been done but were not or areas of nursing care that were done well.
Problem-Solving/ Complexity	The simulation needs to be designed with problem-solving components embedded in the scenario or case that is written. The level of problem-solving needs to be considered (e.g., simple tasks and decisions if students are in a fundamentals course versus more complex problem-solving if students are in an upper-level course and six months from graduating).
Fidelity	A simulation should be designed to be as close an approximation as possible to the real event or activity that is being developed to promote learning. Barrow and Feltovich (1987) suggest that the structure of a realistic, simulated clinical situation requires three elements: 1) relatively little information should be available initially; 2) students should be allowed to investigate freely, employing questions in any sequence; and 3) students get important clinical information over time during the simulation.
Guided Reflection/ Debriefing	Guided reflection reinforces the positive aspects of the experience and encourages reflective learning, which allows the participant to link theory to practice and research, think critically, and discuss how to intervene professionally in complex situations (Bruce, Bridges, & Holcomb, 2003; Jenkins & Turick-Gibson, 1999; Jones, Cason & Mancini, 2002; O'Conner, Albert & Thomas,1999; Rauen, 2001). At the end of the session, the group should discuss the process, outcome, and application of the scenario to clinical practice and review the relevant teaching points (Rauen). Jenkins and Turick-Gibson discuss how the last step in their simulation activity was to share and generalize information with the students.

The Simulation Design Scale (SDS) is a 20-item tool with subscales measuring various design features. Examples of items in the SDS are provided in Table 7-2. The learner completes the tool after participating in a simulation. The design features rated by the learners include objectives/information, student support, problem solving/complexity, fidelity, and guided reflection/debriefing. These features are postulated by Jeffries (2005) as integral to positive learning outcomes in a simulation. Content validity of the instrument was determined by a panel of nine nurse experts. Cronbach's alpha was computed to assess internal consistency and reliability for each scale. The coefficient alpha for the overall scale was 0.94.

Table 7-2. Sample Items from the Simulation Design Scale (SDS)						
Component	Sample Items	5 SA	4 A	3 N	2 D	1 SD
Objectives/ Information	I clearly understood the purpose and objectives of the simulation.					
	The cues were appropriate and geared to promote my understanding.					
Student Support	My need for help was recognized.					
	I was supported in the learning process.					
Problem Solving/ Complexity	I was encouraged to explore all possibilities during the simulation.					
	The simulation provided me with an opportunity to set goals for the patient.					
Fidelity	The scenario resembled a real-life situation.					
Guided Reflection/ Debriefing	Feedback provided was constructive.					

The Implementation Phase

When simulations are implemented, particular components need to be included to ensure a good learning experience, student satisfaction, and good performance by the learners. According to Chickering and Gamson (1987), incorporating principles of best practice in education helps educators implement quality teaching activities and improve student learning. Educational practices are considered a very important component of the learning environment. To measure this component, the Educational Practices Simulation Scale (EPSS) was developed (see Table 7-3). The EPSS is a 16-item tool that the learner completes after a simulation. This tool measures the extent to which principles of best practice in education are being used in simulations although, as a result of factor analysis, the original seven principles (Chickering & Gamson) have been collapsed into four factors. The elements being evaluated in the EPSS scale are active learning, diverse ways of learning, high expectations, and collaboration. The questionnaire was tested for validity and reliability. The content validity was established through a review by nine nurse experts. The coefficient alpha, Cronbach's alpha, was 0.92. Table 7-4 provides sample items from the EPSS which reflect each of the four educational practices.

Table 7-3. Educational Practices in Simulation Scale (EPSS): Components		
Components	**Description**	**Examples**
Active Learning	Through simulation, learners are directly engaged in the activity and obtain immediate feedback and reinforcement of learning. Learning activities can range from simple to complex. Case scenarios, simulation of real-life clinical problems requiring assessment and decision-making skills, role-playing with actors, and critiquing one's or a peer's videotape of a selected skill performance are examples of methods faculty can use to promote active learning (Cioffi, 2001; Lee & Lamp, 2003; Morton, 1996; Nehring, Lashley, & Ellis, 2002; Vandrey & Whitman, 2001). Such active and interactive learning environments encourage students to make connections between concepts and engage them in the learning process.	In a case scenario in which an intubated patient is restless, agitated, and coughing, affecting his oxygenation status, students can be asked to select the most appropriate intervention and describe the rationale for the intervention. The patient simulator can support more complex active learning strategies, since the opportunity allows students to assess a critical health incident (e.g., collapsed lung or status asthmaticus) through the measurement of physiological parameters and communication with the "patient," on-the-spot planning for quick and appropriate nursing interventions, and real-time response by the simulator for realistic evaluation and further intervention (Nehring et al.).
Diverse Ways of Learning	Simulations should be designed to accommodate diverse learning styles and teaching methods and allow students and groups with varying cultural backgrounds to benefit from the experience.	Design a scenario that has visual, auditory, and kinesthetic components. For example, use a monitor or lab reports (visual), program a patient simulator conversation about his symptoms (auditory), and require a procedure to be done (kinesthetic).
High Expectations	High teacher expectations are important for students during a learning experience because expecting students to do well becomes a self-fulfilling prophecy. Students should set goals with faculty and seek advice on how to achieve those goals. When both faculty and students have high expectations for the simulation process and the outcomes, positive results can be achieved.	Set up a scenario with multi-faceted patient problems for the learner who needs to be challenged and needs to advance to the next level of knowledge and skills. Vandrey and Whitman assert that nurses can be pushed to expand their competency levels and empowered to achieve greater learning in a safe learning environment.
Collaboration	Collaboration is pairing students in a simulation to work together. Roles are assigned so that students jointly confirm assessments, make decisions about interventions, and evaluate outcomes.	An example of collaboration is assigning a student the role of primary nurse and a third-year medical student the role of primary physician. Place the two students in a setting where they will be confronted with a deteriorating patient for whom decisions need to be made, interventions need to be performed immediately, and assessments need to be done quickly and accurately.

Table 7-4. Sample Items from the Educational Practices in Simulation Scale (EPSS)						
Component	Sample Items	5 SA	4 A	3 N	2 D	1 SD
Active Learning	I actively participated in the debriefing session after the simulation.					
	I received cues during the simulation in a timely manner.					
Diverse Ways of Learning	The simulation offered a variety of ways in which to learn the material.					
High Expectations	The objectives for the simulation experience were clear and easy to understand.					
Collaboration	I had the chance to work with my peers during the simulation.					

The Outcomes Phase

Simulation technologies used to measure both process and outcomes range from case studies and standardized patients (such as Objective Structured Clinical Exams or OSCEs) to task trainers and high-fidelity human simulators. Formative outcome measures and assessments are situations in which the simulation is used by the learner and/or faculty to mark progress toward personal, course, or program learning goals. Summative evaluations and assessments include determining course competencies, licensing and certification examinations, credentialing processes, and employment decisions (Jeffries, Hovancsek, & Clochesy, 2005). As with any type of assessment, issues of validity and reliability must be considered (Boulet, Murray, Kras, Woodhouse, McAllister, & Ziv, 2003; Clauser, Kane, & Swanson, 2002). A few of the most common outcomes studies will be described.

Knowledge.

According to Schoolcraft and Novotny (2000), knowledge outcomes fall within the cognitive realm and include application, analysis, and synthesis of specified knowledge. To evaluate if the learner has achieved knowledge outcomes, faculty might use verbal questioning or concept/mind mapping (Billings & Halstead). In verbal questioning, the educator asks specific questions that provide an opportunity for the learner to demonstrate understanding of concepts and explain the rationale for her/his actions. With concept/mind mapping, the learner is asked to create a visual display of the clinical situation, including connections among concepts. The learner may then be asked to explain the map and expand upon the rationale for the connections.

Another strategy to evaluate knowledge, the written test, is commonly used in nursing. It may be in the form of a pretest/posttest, posttest only, or pretest/posttest/one week posttest. According to Bloom's taxonomy (Yoder, 1993), multiple-choice knowledge exams can be written to assess different levels of knowledge attainment, including analysis, synthesis, and application. The higher the level, the more the student has to apply and synthesize the knowledge gained.

Skill performance.

A simulation experience or laboratory is an ideal setting for students to develop psychomotor skills without risk of inflicting harm to patients. Becoming comfortable and competent with technology usually requires repeated exposure to that technology, and this is easily accomplished in the simulated environment. Skills requiring procedural steps are receiving increased attention because of their importance to patient care and because of the more rigorous competency standards being required by national organizations, credentialing bodies, and certification groups. Several studies evaluating skills using simulators and/or simulations have found that this mode of teaching sometimes leads to quicker acquisition of the skill than conventional training methods (Ost, DeRosiers, Britt, Fein, Lesser, & Mehta, 2001). Simulation experiences also allow for the use of checklists as measures of skill competencies (Jones, Cason, & Mancini).

Learner satisfaction.

Many educational researchers have been interested in learner satisfaction because if students are satisfied with their learning, their performance is higher (Chickering & Gamson). Simulation activities can be evaluated using quantitative or qualitative measures of students' responses to the experience. Engum, et al., Jeffries et al. (2003), and Johnson et al., all asked students to rate various aspects of an interactive computer experience on 5-6 point Likert scale. Overall, the studies showed that the students were very satisfied with this learning experience. Typical responses were that the experience provided opportunities to "think on your feet," "apply critical thinking skills," and "realize how much I really knew." Similarly, qualitative results from junior and senior students using a human birthing simulator expressed satisfaction in open-ended questions. They reported that they enjoyed having "to work through steps" and "prioritizing" and that the experience seemed "real life."

Critical thinking.

Some of the most common outcomes measures described in the simulation literature have been for critical thinking. Although the measure has varied across studies, most have found that critical thinking does occur (Bruce et al.; Chau et al.; Jenkins

& Turick-Gibson; Johnson et al.; Peterson & Bechtel; Rauen; Ravert; Weis & Guyton-Simmons, 1998). Many studies used Facione and Facione's CCTST (Chau et al.) or CCTDI (Ravert), or an instructor-developed critical thinking inventory and student journals (Jenkins & Turick-Gibson) to assess students' critical thinking abilities. Measuring critical thinking is of interest to nurse educators since this is an essential critical behavior in most nursing curricula. Other concepts that parallel critical thinking and are being explored by nursing educator researchers include clinical diagnostic reasoning, clinical reasoning, and other concepts of higher order of thinking.

Self-confidence.

Studies have shown that simulations can equip learners with skills that can be directly transferred into the clinical setting leading to increased self-confidence and improved clinical judgments (Aronson et al.; Cioffi; Johnson et al.; Peterson & Bechtel; Thiele et al.). Researchers have found that placing students in a realistic clinical simulation to problem-solve and critically-think increases their ability to demonstrate these behaviors (Johnson et al.). Bramble suggested that structured simulations encourage students to think rather than simply memorize facts.

SUMMARY

Simulations require evaluation of many variables, including the simulation design, the implementation process, and learning outcomes. As more simulations are incorporated into nursing curricula and increased research provides greater direction for use of selected clinical models and innovative teaching and learning strategies, nurse educators must carefully analyze the data collected for use in improving future learning using simulations. Nurse educators also need to decide upon the extent to which simulations should play a part in the educational process, particularly clinical teaching and practice. Will simulations become a required part of clinical teaching and learning? Will simulations provide additional opportunities to extend learning in collaborative ways with other health care disciplines? Whatever the final consensus is, the need to teach decision-making and problem-solving skills to nursing students will lead to a continuing increase in the use of simulations in nursing education.

REFERENCES

Aronson, B., Rosa, J., Anfinson, J., & Light, N. (1997). A simulated clinical problem-solving experience. *Nurse Educator, 22*(6), 17-19.

Barrow, H. S., & Feltovich, P. J. (1987). The clinical reasoning process. *Medical Education,, 21*(2), 86-91.

Billings, D. M., & Halstead, J. A. (2005). *Teaching in nursing: A guide for faculty.* (2nd ed.) Philadelphia: W.B. Saunders

Boulet, J. R., Murray, D., Kras, J., Woodhouse, J., McAllister, J., & Ziv, A. (2003). Reliability and validity of a simulation-based acute care skills assessment for medical students and residents. *Anesthesiology,, 99,* 1270-1280.

Bourke, M., & Ihrke, B. (2005). The evaluation process. In D. Billings & J. Halstead (Eds.), *Teaching in nursing: A guide for faculty* (2nd ed.) (pp. 443-464). Philadelphia: W. B. Saunders.

Bramble, K. (1994). Nurse practitioner education: Enhancing performance through the use of the Objective Structured Clinical Assessment. *Journal of Nursing Education, 33*(2), 59-65.

Bruce, S., Bridges, E. J., & Holcomb, J. B. (2003). Preparing to respond: Joint Trauma Training Center and USAF Nursing Warskills Simulation Laboratory. *Critical Care Nursing Clinics of North America, 15,* 149-152.

Chau, J., Chang, A., Lee, I., Ip, W., Lee, D., & Wootton, Y. (2001). Effects of using video-taped vignettes on enhancing students' critical thinking ability in a baccalaureate nursing programme. *Journal of Advanced Nursing, 36*(1), 112-119.

Chickering, A. W., & Gamson, Z. F. (1987, March). Seven principles of good practice in undergraduate education. *AAHE Bulletin, 39*(7), 5-10.

Cioffi, J. (2001). Clinical simulations: Development and validation. *Nurse Education Today, 21,* 477-486.

Clauser, B., Kane, M., & Swanson, D. (2002). Validity issues for performance-based tests scored with computer-automated scoring systems. *Applied Measurement in Education, 15,* 413-432.

Engum, S., Jeffries, P. R., & Fisher, L. (2003). Intravenous catheter training system: Computer-based education versus traditional learning methods. *American Journal of Surgery, 186*(1), 67-74.

Facione N.C., & Facione P.A. (1996). Assessment design issues for evaluating critical thinking in nursing. *Holistic Nursing Practice, 10*(3), 41-53.

Hample, J., Herbold, N., Schneider, M., & Sheeley, A. (1999). Using standardized patients to train and evaluate dietetics students. Journal of the American Dietetic Association, 99(9), 1094-1097.

Jeffries, P.R. (2005). A framework for designing, implementing, and evaluating simulations used as teaching strategies in nursing. Nursing Education Perspectives, 26(2), 28-35.

Jeffries, P., Childs, J., Decker, S., Horn, M., Hovancsek, M., Childress, R., Rogers, K., Feken, C., Spunt, D., & Politi, R. (2004, October 1). How to design, implement, and evaluate simulations in nursing used as a teaching strategy. Presented at the National League for Nursing's Education Summit, Orlando, FL,

Jeffries, P. R., Hovancsek, M. T., & Clochesy, J. M. (2005). Using clinical simulations in distance education. In J. Novotny & R. Davis (Eds.), Distance education in nursing (2nd ed.) (pp. 83-99). New York: Springer Publishing.

Jeffries, P. R., Woolf, S., & Linde, B. (2003). Technology-based vs. traditional instruction: A comparison of two methods for teaching the skill of performing a 12-lead ECG. Nursing Education Perspectives, 24(2), 70-74.

Jenkins, P., & Turick-Gibson, T. (1999). An exercise in critical thinking using role playing. Nurse Educator, 24(6), 11-14.

Johnson, J. H., Zerwic, J. J., & Theis, S. L. (1999). Clinical simulation laboratory: An adjunct to clinical teaching. Nurse Educator, 24(5), 37-41.

Jones, T., Cason, C., & Mancini, M. (2002). Evaluating nurse competency: Evidence of validity for a skills recredentialing program. Journal of Professional Nursing, 18(1), 22-28.

Lee, C., & Lamp, J. (2003). The use of humor and role-playing in reinforcing key concepts. Nurse Educator, 28(2), 61-62.

Lincoln, Y. S., & Guba, E. G. (1985). Naturalistic inquiry. Beverly Hills, CA: Sage.

Morgan, P. J., & Cleave-Hogg, D. (2000). Evaluation of medical students' performance using the anesthesia simulator. Medical Education, 34, 42-45.

Morton, P. G. (1996). Using a critical care simulation laboratory to teach students. Critical Care Nurse, 17(6), 66-69.

Nehring, W. M., Lashley, F. A., & Ellis, W. E. (2002). Critical incident nursing management using human patient simulators. Nursing Education Perspectives, 23(3), 128-132.

O'Connor, F., Albert, M., & Thomas, M. (1999). Incorporating standardized patients into a psychosocial nurse practitioner program. Archives of Psychiatric Nursing, 8(5), 240-247.

Oermann, M. H., & Gaberson, K. B. (2006). *Evaluation and testing in nursing education* (2nd ed.). New York: Springer Publishing.

Ost, D., DeRosiers, E., Britt, J., Fein, A., Lesser, M., & Mehta, A. (2001). Assessment of a bronchoscopy simulator. *American Journal of Respiratory and Critical Care Medicine, 164*, 2248-2255.

Peterson, M., & Bechtel, G. (2000). Combining the arts: An applied critical thinking approach in the skills laboratory. *Nursing Connections, 13*(2), 43-49.

Polit, D. F., & Hungler, B. P. (1995). *Nursing research: Principles and methods*. Philadelphia: J. B. Lippincott.

Rauen, C. A. (2001). Using simulation to teach critical thinking skills. *Critical Care Nursing Clinics of North America, 13*(1), 93-103.

Ravert, P. (2002). An integrative review of computer based simulation in the education process. *CIN: Computers, Informatics, Nursing, 20*(5), 203-208.

Robertson, B. (2006). An obstetric simulation experience in an undergraduate nursing curriculum. *Nurse Educator, 31*(2), 74-78.

Schoolcraft, V., & Novotny, J. (2000). *A nuts-and-bolts approach to teaching nursing*. New York: Springer Publishing.

Stufflebeam, D.L., & Webster, W.J. (1994). An analysis of alternative approaches to evaluation. In J.S. Stark & A. Thomas (Eds.), *Assessment and program evaluation* (pp. 331-348). Needham Heights, MA: Simon & Schuster.

Thiele, J., Holloway, J., Murphy, D., Pardavis, J., & Stuckey, M. (1991). Perceived and actual decision making by novice baccalaureate students. *Western Journal of Nursing Research, 13*, 616-626.

Vandrey, C., & Whitman, M. (2001). Simulator training for novice critical care nurses. *American Journal of Nursing, 101*(9), 24GG-24LL.

Weis, P., & Guyton-Simmons, J. (1998). A computer simulation for teaching critical thinking skills. *Nurse Educator, 23*(2), 30-33.

Weller, J. M. (2004). Simulation in undergraduate medical education: Bridging the gap between theory and practice. *Medical Education, 38*, 32-38.

Winston, I., & Szarek, J. L. (2005). Problem-based learning using a human patient simulator. *Medical Education, 39*(5), 526-527.

Winters, J., Hauck, B., Riggs, J., Clawson, J., & Collins, J. (2003). Use of videotaping to assess competencies and course outcomes. *Journal of Nursing Education, 42*(10), 472-476.

Yoder, M. E. (1993). Computer use and nursing research: Transfer of cognitive learning to a clinical skill: Linear versus interactive video. *Western Journal of Nursing Research, 15*, 115-117.

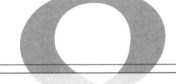

CHAPTER 8

SETTING UP A SIMULATION LABORATORY

Debra L. Spunt, MS, RN, FAAN

*"The essence of education is not to stuff you with
facts but to help you discover your uniqueness,
to teach you how to develop it,
and then to show you how to give it away."*

Leo Buscaglia

The simulation center, according to Infante (1985), is a replication of a clinical setting that allows the learner the opportunity to integrate theory and practice, think critically, and ensure patient safety. This environment is referred to by many names: skills lab, nursing lab, learning resources center (LRC), learning center, and clinical simulation lab (CSL). One of the primary roles of the CSL is to serve as a resource to faculty and students during the development, implementation and evaluation of simulation activities. This chapter will focus on the physical learning environment and the function of a simulation center, which includes space, supplies, organization and flexibility of the environment, technology support, and equipment.

SPACE

The allocation of space reflects the institution's commitment, need, and resources. However large or small, the CSL space should be able to accommodate multiple teaching and evaluation strategies (e.g., formal demonstrations, return demonstrations, small groups, and self-directed learning activities) that are selected, based on desired learning outcomes. The identification of potential teaching approaches will determine the exact needs of each lab (deTornyay & Thompson, 1987).

With the teaching strategies identified, the design phase of lab development begins by assembling an interdisciplinary planning and design team. The team should consist of the dean or senior administration, facilities manager, faculty, simulation specialist, architect, technology consultant, and audiovisual (AV) consultant. The design team will need to keep several concerns in mind as they develop the plan for new space or renovation of existing space. Once the team has agreed upon the needs and a general plan, the architect will provides a detailed space-by-space plan. The sample plan in Table 8-1 describes new or existing space to be used for a medical/surgical simulation lab. The plan includes the following:

- quantity and type(s) of simulation space needed
- how and by whom the space will be used
- location in building and adjacent spaces (e.g., rest room, elevator — passenger vs. freight)
- support and other ancillary spaces (e.g., storage, office)
- equipment and infrastructures needed to support learning
- special features (e.g., size of door, linoleum or tile, lights — dimmer, module...)

Table 8-1. Sample Medical/Surgical Lab Plan

Classification	Description
Function	Various medical/surgical lab stations around the perimeter of the room where students can work in small groups of 3 or 4 and center seating for classroom instruction and demonstration. Includes combination nursing/teaching station.
Relationship	Locate near faculty for students to review their work and provide direct access to general circulation as well as clean lab storage, dirty lab storage, student pack storage, and simulation model/equipment storage.
New Equipment – Built-in	• Ceiling track for patient lift transport over each set of 4 beds • 2 hand washing stations with goose neck style faucet, 1-hand and 1-knee controls • Motorized projection screen, 8'x 8', to close flush with the ceiling surface • Whiteboard, 4' x 8', non-glare • Digitizing tablet wallboard • Ceiling-mounted color TV receivers/monitors connected into playback system • Wall-mounted over each bed: Headwall unit with multiple live electrical outlets and gas valves (functioning with simulated oxygen and vacuum at 50mmHg), safety equipment-glove and sharps box • Wall clocks with second hand • A nurses' station … The front part of this station consists of an instructor's table lectern that contains a state-of-the-art PC with overhead projection capability, a ½" VHS recorder with video projection, and sound capability; an upholstered chair, and under-counter cabinetry that can be designed in a U-shape (_ /) configuration to make the area wheelchair accessible. At the rear of the nurses' station are upper and lower cabinets, the latter of which have a sink, space for a computer, and space for a computerized medication administration system (e.g., OMNICELL).
New Equipment – Movable	• 8 bed areas (4 on each side of the room) with bedside computer and chair (with arms that can double as a bedside chair for patient transfers). Each bed area should have an over-bed table, and a bedside table. • 11 mar-resistant tables and 18 ergonomic (stackable) chairs. At least one student station must be wheelchair accessible.
Existing Equipment	• None
Utilities	• Compressed air with vacuum • Zoned lighting over each bed with individual bed switch and lighting on a dimmer switch over the teaching area • Multiple electrical outlets (quads) • 2 Ethernet connections at instructor's station • Provide audio, voice, and data outlets at lecture station connected to building and campus networks. Include two voice and data service outlet jacks additionally, along with three video transmission/reception jacks where directed, and convenience outlets spaced 12' on center.
Special Requirements	• Vinyl tile floor and acoustical ceiling with sound insulation • Accessible, flexible system to supply current and future power, data, voice, and video connections • Lighting dimmer with blackout and separate switching between instructor's station area and seating • Hospital doors/dual leaf with vision panel with shade NOTE: Lights should be zoned to allow front lights and houselights to be controlled separately to achieve lighting levels that are acceptable for note taking. If incandescent lights are used, the controls should be dimmers. If fluorescent lights are used, cut-out switches are needed to allow a minimum number of tubes to be left on for note taking during projection. There should be no dimmers on fluorescent lights.

The actual space allocation for the CSL will be determined by the anticipated use by students and members of the community. Regardless of whether the CSL space is located in an academic building or in a renovated hospital/clinical structure, several considerations are critical if teaching and learning are to be enhanced. The space should be column-free with good ventilation, flexible illumination, functioning plumbing, and ample electrical outlets (each outlet should include 4 taps). The space should be easily accessible and have doors at least four feet wide. It should have external and internal corridors at least eight feet wide to allow for the movement of equipment, storage space, and some type of security system. The technology infrastructure needs to include access to and interaction with the institution's computer systems, and a plan should be in place to support and regularly update all computerized educational simulation programs needed for teaching and learning.

The actual design of the CSL can be as basic as a bed and over-bed table, or as complex as a fully functional critical care unit with monitors, suction, and power columns. On average, a teaching unit or bed station should be approximately 85 square feet, a space that is large enough to allow up to 4 students to work together. Figure 8-1 provides a diagram of how a teaching unit can be arranged.

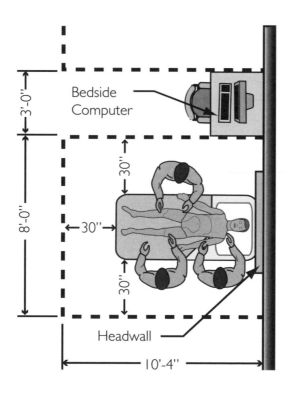

Figure 8-1.
Simulated Teaching Unit

The actual layout of the total lab will depend on how the lab will be used; it will take on one configuration if it will be used for teaching, another if it will be used for evaluation. The type of learning and the level of the learner also will influence the design of the lab space. The lab may reflect a clinical specialty such as home care, perioperative nursing, or maternal nursing. Some labs are multifocus in order to include many clinical specialties in one space (see Figure 8-2). Frequently seen combinations include pediatrics and maternity nursing and medical/surgical and health assessment labs. If the lab is to be used to teach physical assessment, the space will need to be designed to ensure privacy during practice sessions by including ceiling tracks appropriate for the installation of privacy curtains or adequate space for portable screens. The latter may require increased floor space and storage space. Additional space modifications may be required to accommodate the needs of several teachers, or of diverse students. Space modifications also may vary based on the teaching/evaluation methods and the number of individuals using the lab at any one time.

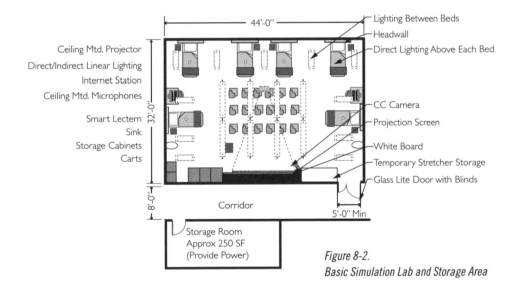

Figure 8-2.
Basic Simulation Lab and Storage Area

A separate control room for evaluation of individuals or groups of students will need to include particular specifications both in the lab and the control room area (see Figure 8-3). The average space requirement for a 1-2 bed lab of this type is usually 500 sq. ft. with a control room of 150 sq. ft. The control room usually has a one-way window into the lab, which allows for a full view of the room by the faculty, observers (students), and technician if one is needed. The lighting in the outer lab should consist of fluorescent lights over the bed and throughout the room. Natural lighting should be avoided in this area because it can affect the quality of recorded events. Cameras should have a wide-angle lens and be wall- or ceiling-mounted with camera control (zoom and wide angle) from the control room. The recording equipment can be as simple as a VCR or as complex as a system with a digital uptake feed and sound mixer for audio quality. In order to capture audio of the event, microphones need to be mounted in the ceiling.

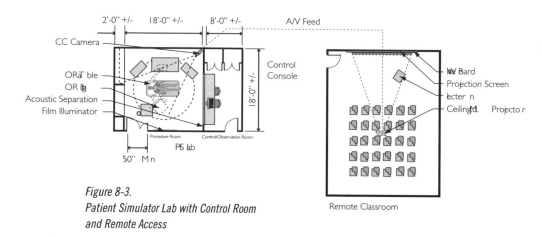

Figure 8-3.
Patient Simulator Lab with Control Room
and Remote Access

Because the microphones will be ceiling-mounted, it is essential that the ventilation system for this room be very quiet and that walls are made of a soundproof material. If cost is a factor, wireless microphones and walkie-talkies can be used. A simulation of a clinical encounter may be electronically viewed in a remote classroom during a live classroom session, adding to the integration of didactic material to a clinical situation as depicted in Figure 8-3. Faculty, students, or actors may participate in the encounter. Examples of this type of teaching strategy are an interview with a schizophrenic patient, assessment of a post-operative patient upon return from surgery and 24 hours post-surgery, and a developmental assessment of a child.

A very important aspect of space allocation is the need for adequate storage and equipment preparation areas in and immediately adjacent to the CSL. Like the simulation labs themselves, the storage area needs to be well ventilated, well illuminated, and have electrical services, running water and some type of security system, especially if syringes, needles, and sutures are stored in this area. The storage and prep space must be large enough to hold both durable and disposable equipment, task trainers, and full size mannequins. The suggested space for storage is 250 sq. ft. for every 1200 sq. ft. of simulation lab space. Lockable cabinets in this area provide for a safe, enclosed space for the storage of disposable, electrical, and sensitive equipment. Wire, metal, or wooden shelf units that are sturdy and have extra wide shelves (at least 24 inches deep) are appropriate for the storage of mannequins, simulators, and task trainers in individual carrying cases. In addition to storage, this area will be used for equipment maintenance, repair, and setup. A table or tabletop shelf – with direct lighting and extra electrical outlets, and adjacent to a deep sink – is ideal for cleaning and draining equipment. IV arms and the mannequin bladders need to be drained and flushed on a regular basis. This shelf over the sink can hold cleaning supplies and hooks to hang equipment and allows for adequate drainage of mannequin parts.

EQUIPMENT

The careful selection of both durable and disposable equipment will enhance the ability to simulate real clinical situations. All equipment selected should be in good operating condition and reflect current technology. The use of out-of-date durable equipment makes it difficult for the learner to transfer skills and knowledge to patient care settings. For example, the use of an old patient-controlled analgesia (PCA) pump, which is no longer manufactured or used, would not be appropriate for simulation even if one could find tubing and the parts to service it. When selecting equipment for purchase, one should look into the possibility of trading in an old model for a new one for a reduced price. Some manufacturers will take older equipment, such as beds and ventilators, clean and refurbish them, and upgrade parts to sell at a reduced price. When selecting the medical/ durable equipment to be purchased, a good way to start is to contact local clinical agencies and request the list of vendors used. Consider the following when selecting equipment for purchase:

- Who will be using the equipment? How often?

- Is this equipment used by a large number of clinical agencies in your area where students have clinical experiences?

- Is the disposable material necessary to the related equipment (e.g., tubing for an intravenous pump or controller) available at a reduced fee or at no cost?

- Are the educational materials available or are there on-site in-service classes so that students and faculty can learn to use the equipment?

- Is the company interested in donating and/or upgrading equipment for the CSL?

Since sophisticated technology will be required, the purchase and maintenance of equipment for the CSL can be expensive and labor intensive. Many CSLs have limited funds and limited technological resources, so the rental, leasing, borrowing, or sharing of equipment often is a viable option to ensure access to specialized equipment when needed.

Durable Equipment

Selecting state-of-the-art durable equipment for purchase can be a little like buying a car: the same basic product is available from many vendors, and there is great benefit to "shopping around." Before purchasing equipment, it is essential to assess the equipment currently in use by local health care agencies. It is helpful to visit such agencies to see how they use the equipment of interest and observe its quality and function in real clinical settings. Contact the agency's purchasing department for purchasing information related to the equipment. Ask for the manufacturer's or distributor's name and contact information, cost of the product, any special contractual agreement (e.g., free tubing) related to the equipment, and reliability of the company. Obtaining this type of information for several vendors who sell the same equipment allows you to do some "comparison shopping." When communicating with a prospective vendor, emphasize the intended use of the equipment and the types of learners (novice students to expert nurses) who will be using the equipment. Also, do not hesitate to ask for a reduced price or a donation and/or some type of creative purchasing agreement (e.g., purchase one item at the regular price and get the second free or at a substantial reduction). After review of all available information related to the equipment to be purchased, follow your institution's policies related to procurement of durable equipment. Keep track of the purchasing request until the equipment is delivered and paid for. Upon delivery, test the equipment with the vendor and ask for an in-service program on the operation and troubleshooting of the equipment. The final step of the purchase process is to keep a file that will provide information on vendor contact information, repairs, replacement, and satisfaction with the entire purchase experience for reference at a later date.

Disposable Equipment

The quantity and type of disposable equipment needed for the CSL will depend on the number of learners and types of learning experience in which they are expected to engage. Disposable equipment can be purchased through medical supply companies or from a clinical agency. It is often economical to arrange for an ongoing purchase agreement with a local hospital and purchase items in bulk rather then buying small quantities from a manufacturer. Purchasing agreements should include the delivery and replacement of damaged goods by the vendor or hospital. Upon delivery, the supplies should be cataloged and stored in a clean, dry area located in or adjacent to the CSL.

A cost-saving alternative is to use out-of-date supplies from vendors. If vendors change a product's name or packaging, they may have disposable supplies that they cannot sell and would be happy to donate to your CSL. The use of these supplies will increase the quantity of available practice supplies without increased cost. These supplies should be clearly labeled as NON-STERILE so that there is no confusion about their status. It might also be helpful to store used and out-of-date items in a clearly marked separate area within the storage room.

Mannequins, Models and Simulators

Completing the CLS will require mannequins, models, and clinical simulators. Table 8-2 lists the different types of simulators used by health care educators. The use of clinical simulators in a well-stocked lab allows for the transformation of the room into a clinical environment. Life-like mannequins, anatomical models, and simulators help develop assessment, problem solving, and critical thinking skills as well as the psychomotor skills necessary to prepare students and health care providers to deliver safe and efficient patient care in multiple health care settings (patient's home, hospital, long-term care center, schools, and business).

Table 8-2. Types of Simulators and Simulations

Type	Definition	Example
Task Trainer	Part of a mannequin designed for a specific psychomotor skill	Ear model, central/PICC line dressing model, Leopold palpation model
Mannequin	Passive full body mannequin with exchangeable parts (e.g., wounds)	Resusci® Anne, age-specific mannequins (baby, geriatric)
Basic Simulator	Full body simulator with installed human qualities (breath sounds, childbirth)	VitalSim™ child and infant, Nursing Anne, Noelle™ birthing simulator
Patient Simulator	Full body simulator that can be programmed to respond to affective and psychomotor changes	SimMan®, Human Patient Simulator™
Computer Assisted Instruction (CAI)	Passive and interactive programmable software	Fetal monitoring, ABG interpretation
Virtual Reality	Complete simulated environment that includes audio, visual, tactile, hardware, electronics, and software	Virtual hospital/nursing home, IV simulator, robotics, data gloves
Standardized Patient (SP)	Individual who is trained to portray a patient or teach students using the SP as a teaching tool	Scenarios related to invasive and non-invasive physical examination, interview, patient education, and discharge planning
Web-based Simulation	Multimedia and interactive information accessed from around the world	Access via hyperlinks to virtual clinical environments in action (e.g., time lapse demonstration of the development of a pressure sore)
Blended Simulation	Use of multiple types of simulation to provide a comprehensive learning experience	SP: interview, simulator: physical examination and intervention, SP: education and discharge planning

Mannequins and clinical simulators can be tailored to meet individual learner needs and teaching goals. As a result of the need for today's clinicians to be able to provide high quality care to a sicker and more diverse population, the number of clinical/assessment simulators used in CSLs has proliferated. These simulators add to the ability of the CSL to replicate various clinical situations and emphasize the critical thinking and prioritization skills needed for decision-making and safe clinical practice. The categories of simulators that seem to be the most realistic and advanced are those related to normal and abnormal health assessment findings (eye, ear, heart and lung sounds, reproductive organs) and cardiovascular interpretations. Health assessment simulators can be used by learners at all levels and from multiple specialties. The beginning nursing student will use the simulator to learn basic assessment skills and to differentiate normal and abnormal findings. Graduate students and practicing health care professionals will use the same simulators for higher-level skills such as diagnosis and appropriate medical/nursing treatment to be prescribed. Simulators used in the area of cardiovascular nursing range from arrhythmia/dysrhythmia interpretation and hemodynamic monitoring to the integration of multiple simulators for the purpose of a "mock code."

Numerous types of task-trainers are used to add to the full-body simulator encounter and enhance psychomotor skill acquisition. The selection of the appropriate simulator is a process of matching the right tool with the right educational objectives. Choosing the correct simulator requires an understanding of the strengths, weaknesses, and limitations of each product, knowledge of the desired learning outcomes, and knowledge of each faculty member's comfort and familiarity with the simulator.

Multiple equipment vendors and manufacturers market the same task trainers and mannequins for health care professionals and use in educational programs. Regardless of the program, there are several factors to consider when purchasing any type of simulator. The faculty and simulation specialist should evaluate the following when purchasing a simulator:

- How durable is this product? Can it be used in a variety of settings? Indoors? Outdoors?

- What is the life expectancy of the mannequin and its movable parts?

- Is a warranty available?

- Will the product be serviced? By whom?

- How long is the product expected to last?

- What is the cost of upgrades — software and hardware?

- Is there any type of special care required for the outer surface of the mannequin (cleaners, adhesive remover)?

Routine care by the faculty, students, and CSL staff will help maintain and extend the life expectancy of the simulator. The following section includes recommendations to maximize the life of your mannequins and task trainers. The outer surface or skin of mannequins is made of vinyl, flexible or rigid plastic, and fabric. The outer surface must be able to tolerate repeated applications of chemicals such as betadine and tincture of benzoin. The surface of any mannequin must be easy to clean with soap and water. Any mannequins on which dressings are applied will need to be cleaned with adhesive remover. Movable parts and limbs are constructed of hard plastic and metal. The joints and other moveable parts are attached using hinges and other bolt and nut devices. In addition to moveable external parts, some mannequins have interchangeable internal parts, which often slide into place via a track and are secured in place with a nut and bolt.

The repair/maintenance and parts replacement of the mannequin will depend on the frequency of use, number and type of moving parts, and the type of simulation skills to be performed. Mannequins used for catheterization and rectal examination may become torn or cracked as a result of frequent internal manipulation. Glue for vinyl and plastic, sutures, and hot pen (the heat from the pen softens the area that can be remolded and/or fused together to make a new, stronger seam) can be used to repair and reinforce weak and high-stress areas. Replaceable parts often are included with the mannequin or available for purchase. Skin and veins can be replaced easily on mannequins used for psychomotor skills like intravenous therapy. As the mannequin's parts become unrepairable or replacement parts are no longer available, one can interchange parts among mannequins or modify the intended use of the mannequin based on its limitations/capabilities. For example, you can use a mannequin with destroyed legs as a bilateral amputee. The mannequin can still be used for tracheotomy care, enteral feedings, and other skills simulation that do not require the lower limbs.

Although expensive, a mannequin will last a long time with proper care and preventive maintenance. Mannequins should be appropriately stored; most manufacturers provide a storage unit for each mannequin at the time of purchase. The common types of storage cases seen today are: soft leather zipper bag with carrying strap; canvas zipper bag; cardboard box with attached or detachable lid; hard plastic box, and hard-sided case. Storage areas must be dry and cool to prevent mannequin damage. An area that is hot and humid may damage internal and external parts. Mildew, mold, spores, and bacteria may grow on and in mannequins even if they are cleaned and thoroughly dried before storage, or if they become wet/damp in the storage area.

SCHEDULING, STAFFING, AND INVENTORY

Clinical Simulation Labs are a major component of most nursing curricula. Yet they are very costly to supply and operate. Careful preplanning, good organization of space, and appropriate use and care of equipment, mannequins, models, simulators, and disposable supplies can enhance the cost effectiveness of the lab(s).

The day-to-day functions of the CSL depend on a preplanned system to maximize the scheduling, supply distribution, and replenishment. A goal of the CSL is to project the schedule and supplies prior to the start of the academic year. But there is no ideal world in the CSL. Extra classes (from within your school, other schools, and health care agencies), students' needs, tours, and presentations for community groups occur without warning. Although there is always an unpredictable aspect of CSL, one can predict most of the supply needs per semester or unit of study.

Record keeping is a key component to smooth operation in the CSL and should include room schedules, tours/presentations/workshops, student data (i.e., all lab sections, open lab attendance, borrowed equipment), supplies needed, supplies used, indicators for supply/equipment replacement, and any additional data specific to your CSL. The CSL documentation process may be paper and pencil, automated, or a combination based on the size of the CSL and computer access.

Requests for scheduling the CSL should be made six months prior to the beginning of the academic semester or unit of study. The faculty coordinating or responsible for the courses requiring lab time should communicate the following information to the CSL coordinator or director:

- Course number and title
- Faculty responsible for lab portion of course
- Phone number/beeper and email address of faculty
- Date request submitted (this helps to prioritize room assignments)
- Day of week, time of day, and dates lab will be needed
- Number of students
- Purpose of lab and any special needs (e.g., AV, ventilator, crash cart, and simulators)
- Detailed list or description of what will be taught in each lab session (this will be used for lab setup)

One example of a lab reservation form that can be submitted in writing or via email, is provided as Figure 8-4.

Figure 8-4, Internal Clinical Simulation Lab (CSL) Reservation Form

Name: _____   Date: _____

Phone Number: _____

Course Number and Faculty:_____

Date(s) Requested: _____

Lab(s) Requested:_____

Purpose: _____

_____

_____

_____

Equipment Needed and Set-up:_____

_____

_____

_____

For Office Use Only

Time Required for Setup_____   Done By _____

Time Required for Breakdown _____   Done By _____

Comments_____

_____

_____

_____

_____

Labs also need to be staffed. Staffing should start with at least one employee whose job or a designated part of his/her job is to manage the day-to-day operation of the lab. Ideally, this individual holds a faculty position within the school and serves as the Lab Director/Manager/Coordinator. This person should understand the curriculum and how the CSL helps faculty meet curriculum goals. Ideally, the CSL Coordinator/Director is a member of the school's curriculum committee and other appropriate committees (e.g., Technology Committee, Learning Resources Center Committee) in order to help faculty integrate simulation into the curriculum. Administrative support is needed for record keeping and ordering. The skills needed and the time commitment related to this position will depend on the size of your CSL.

The actual staffing of the labs for classes and day-to-day functions can be handled in many different ways, but someone should be assigned to the lab to coordinate setup and cleanup of the lab, serve as a resource for students if the school has open lab time, provide remediation for students needing assistance, and assist in recruitment and community activities. Often, faculty will teach a session in the lab but are not part of the CSL staff. The staffing issues reflect the use and mission of the CSL. It is important for discussion to take place around the following questions:

- Do CSL staff teach and evaluate students?
- Do staff assist in scheduled lab sessions and/or serve as resources in open labs?
- Who sets up, cleans up, and stocks the lab?
- Are there academic requirements or limitations related to function of staff members? (e.g., Can a nurse with a BSN evaluate a BSN student?)
- Does the Board of Nursing or other regulatory body specify who can teach/evaluate students and how much clinical time can be in simulation?

The answer to these questions will provide direction for the type and number of staff needed.

Graduate and undergraduate students make excellent employees in the CSL. Employing graduate students as staff in the CSL is beneficial to the school and the graduate students. Graduate students may work as Graduate Teaching Assistants (GTAs) and receive tuition remission, an hourly stipend, flexible hours, and teaching experience. GTAs bring a variety of clinical experience and an interest in learning to the CSL. They are role models to the undergraduate (pre-licensure) students who work in the CSL. Undergraduate students work closely with the GTAs and serve as peer educators. Both types of students share the responsibility of assisting with the day-to-day operation of the CSL (see Table 8-3). If graduate student help is not an option, nurses in the community who are retired, on disability, or looking for work around a flexible schedule may be the answer to your staffing needs. The nurse from the community can teach and evaluate students, assist faculty, and help with the day-to-day operation of the CSL.

Table 8-3. Clinical Simulation Laboratory Staff Job Descriptions

Responsibility	Assistant (Undergraduate Year 1)	Peer Educator (Undergraduate Year 2)	Teaching Assistant (Master's)	Teaching/Research Assistant (Doctoral)
Supplies & Set-up	Labs; rooms; student bins; taking down bins	Labs; rooms; student bins; taking down bins	Assist with lab/ room set-up; assist with bin assembly and take down	Not Applicable
Storeroom	Clean up; stock	Clean up; stock	Assist with clean up and stock	Not Applicable
Validation	Set up rooms; document scores; start students for validation	Set up rooms; document scores; start students for validation	Set up rooms; document scores; start students for validation	Review videos; grade videos; counsel students after validation
Open Labs	Resource person	Resource person	Demonstration; resource person	Demonstration; resource person
Skills Labs	Set up students for skills	Set up students for skills; sign off on all except EKG	Set up students for skills; sign off skills	Sign off skills
Scheduled Labs & Tours	Participate with recruitment activities	Participate with recruitment activities	Assigned to lab; resource; participate with recruitment activities	Assigned to faculty; mentor relationship with faculty; participate with recruitment activities
Research	Not applicable	Not applicable	Not applicable	Data collection; data analysis; report writing
Presentations	Not applicable	Not applicable	Not applicable	Collaborative preparation and presentation of findings

INVENTORY AND RESTOCKING

The volume of equipment, supplies, and transactions that are needed for the day-to-day operation of a CSL necessitate a structured record-keeping program. The inventory system can be written or automated (e.g., barcode system or spreadsheet). A planned system will save time and increase accuracy in supply distribution and acquisition. Ideally, a system would provide cross referencing, automatic notification of low inventory items, notification of routine equipment maintenance/calibration, and generation of reports. No matter what format is selected, one must be able to retrieve information about equipment, mannequins, models, simulators, supplies needed for particular lab sections or units, supplies actually used, and quantity available in storage.

Keeping track of disposable supplies to be used and those actually used can be one of the most difficult and time-consuming aspects of the functioning of the CSL. The inventory of this equipment can either be formatted by skill (e.g., tracheotomy care), by the type of equipment (sterile gauze pads, 2x2's, 4x4's), or cross references that allow one to change the format based on the need at the time (e.g., lab setup or review of total equipment available per category). An inventory system spreadsheet contains the item name, its description, its location in the CSL, its cost and how it is available for purchase (individual, box, case), and where and how to order supplies (hospital central supply, supply vendor). The system also should be able to provide an accurate inventory of supplies on hand, thus preventing the labor-intensive process of counting every item prior to reordering.

Durable equipment, mannequins, models, and simulators do not to need to be replaced on a regular basis, but must be kept current and in working order. The estimated lifespan for each type of durable equipment differs based on the item. Beds last longer than stethoscopes; therefore, do not use a universal lifespan formula for all durable products. Setting up the process can take quite a bit of time. However, once it is established, you need only to revise it if the cost or student numbers change dramatically and/or when you add a new product to inventory. The following formula is used to determine the per usage value of a durable item:

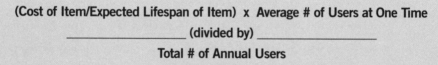

(Cost of Item/Expected Lifespan of Item) x Average # of Users at One Time
_____ **(divided by)** _____
Total # of Annual Users

For example, a new bed might cost $2500.00, and it should last at least 25 years. If student lab groups average 8 students per session and the average annual enrollment per year is 700 students, then the per usage value of a bed is $1.14 [(2500 / 25) x 8] / 700). By comparison, a stethoscope costs $125.00 and should last 5 years. The per usage value of a stethoscope for these same students is $0.29 [(125/5) x 8] / 700)

The inventory format for durable equipment should include the following: type of equipment (beds, power columns), manufacturer information (name, vendor, and phone numbers), serial number, cost, and location in CSL. The consolidation of this information provides quick and easy access for repair, replacement, education, and newly released equipment from a particular manufacturer. Annual budget projections are achieved using the CSL data inventory database, which holds information on all products used in the lab, durable and consumable cost, and number used for each lab event. The data can be used to report information such as the following:

- cost per student
- cost per group of students
- cost per course
- cost per program (e.g., RN, LPN)

The reports can be exported to a spreadsheet, and charts and graphs can be generated to compare annual expenses.

SUMMARY

Fidelity or realism is one of the key design characteristics that should be included in every simulation (Jeffries, 2005). This chapter emphasizes the key components of the simulation environment necessary to enhance the teaching strategy and the students' ability to achieve the desired curriculum outcomes. The selection of equipment, supplies, and simulators is integral to bringing the vision alive and transforming the lab environment into a realistic replication of a clinical setting. The successful day-to-day operation and management of the lab also determine the effectiveness of the CSL.

CONCLUSION

The design of a simulation area that realistically reflects the clinical practice environment will help prepare students for safer and more efficient practice. Faced with the challenges of today's health care environment, nurse educators must explore innovative ways to teach nursing students about the real world of nursing in a cost-effective, efficient, and high-quality manner. The simulated environment provides a setting in which the student can actively engage in the learning process and receive feedback from faculty. The CSL that has been designed with the right blend of simulators allows students to learn and practice in an environment where mistakes result in teachable moments. The simulation lab fosters learning, not anxiety (Hanson, 1993). Clinical simulation, combined with clinical experience and other teaching methods, is a powerful tool to prepare competent nurses for clinical nursing practice (Morton, 1996).

REFERENCES

deTornyay, R., & Thompson, M. A. (1987). *Strategies for teaching nursing* (3rd ed.). New York: Delmar.

Hanson, G. F. (1993). Refocusing the skills laboratory. *Nurse Educator, 18*(2), 10-12.

Infante, M. S. (1985). *The clinical laboratory in nursing education* (2nd ed.). New York: Wiley.

Jeffries, P. R. (2005). A framework for designing, implementing, and evaluating simulations used as teaching strategies in nursing. *Nursing Education Perspectives, 26*(2), 96-103.

Morton, P. G. (1996). Using a critical care simulation laboratory to teach students. *Critical Care Nurse, 17*(6), 66-69.

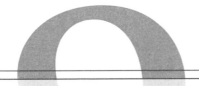

CHAPTER 9
USING COLLABORATION TO ENHANCE THE EFFECTIVENESS OF SIMULATED LEARNING IN NURSING EDUCATION

Reba Moyer Childress, MSN, APRN-BC, FNP, Pamela R. Jeffries, DNS, RN, FAAN, & Cheryl Feken Dixon, MS, RN

"Part of teaching is helping students learn how to
tolerate ambiguity, consider possibilities,
and ask questions that are unanswerable."

Sara Lawrence Lightfoot

Nursing, like many other professions, has used diverse educational methods to guide students' learning and help them be effective in practice. Most of the methods are teacher-centered and focus primarily on the cognitive domain (e.g., lectures, seminars, discussions). However, faculty are challenged to find more effective ways to prepare students to care for patients who are more acutely ill, to manage the care of increasing numbers of patients, and to practice in high-tech, fast-paced clinical environments. Therefore, new ways must be found to help faculty meet these challenges. Simulation in health care education is evolving into one of the most effective ways to facilitate students' acquisition of psychomotor skills, decision making skills, and skills related to collaborating with other health care team members (Loyd, Lake, & Greenberg, 2004).

With the advancement of technology, the demands on health care providers have become more complex (Koerner, 2003; Long, 2004). Health care providers face increasingly complex patient care situations, the need to make decisions rapidly in spite of conflicting or incomplete information, and the need to collaborate more effectively among members of the health care team (Hamman, 2004; Maddox, Wakefield, & Bull, 2001). Such realities challenge nurse educators and others in the health professions to design teaching, learning, and evaluation strategies that enhance students' abilities to practice safely and effectively in this health care environment. Among the strategies suggested to assist educators in meeting student learning needs and developing their practice competencies are e-learning, virtual reality, and scenario-based simulation (Koerner; Ziv, Wolpe, Small, & Glick, 2003). The use of collaborative learning using scenario-based simulation holds exceptional promise for education, particularly for the education of nurses.

This chapter defines collaborative learning in a health care simulation environment, describes different types of collaborative learning experiences that can be incorporated into a simulation, describes roles faculty may play when designing a simulation with an emphasis on collaboration, and discusses benefits and challenges associated with incorporating collaborative learning in a simulated environment.

COLLABORATIVE LEARNING DEFINED

Collaborative learning in a simulated health care environment is the process of individuals functioning together as a group for the purpose of acquiring knowledge and skills to improve patient outcomes. Working together results in greater understanding that would not have occurred had each person worked independently. Team members are assigned to or assume various roles, have a common objective, and function in a virtual health care setting to achieve common goals (Gokhale, 1995). Through interactive experiences both in and beyond the classroom, collaborative learners become aware of relationships between interactions and understanding.

ESTABLISHING A COLLABORATIVE LEARNING ENVIRONMENT

In all disciplines, learning involves induction into the intellectual culture of the discipline (Hamilton, 1997). For example, to understand anthropology, students need to learn how anthropologists look at people and events. In order to enact the role of a historian, anthropologist, physician, or nurse, students need appropriate information, language, and experiences. Also, opportunities need to be developed through which learners can connect the information, language, and experiences to their own knowledge and experience to ensure that there is understanding, not merely an accumulation of knowledge.

Lectures, laboratory courses, and videos are learning tools that foster efficient and rapid delivery of essential information or development of specialized skills or techniques. However, unless students apply this knowledge and these skills to the context of work done by individuals in the field, the skills, knowledge, and information may be forgotten. As students are involved in problem-solving and decision-making situations similar to those faced by health care professionals, they need to integrate information, language, and skills into action and dialogue. As students become immersed in this type of learning environment, they can solve problems together and gain a better understanding of roles and responsibilities specific to each discipline.

Deciding when to use collaborative learning is dependent upon the nature of the knowledge and understanding expected in a particular area. Facts, standardized skills, and interventions are efficiently learned in a lecture format. Application of new information and new skills in response to less predictable real-life situations is more effectively accomplished in a collaborative atmosphere in which students can interact and integrate knowledge and skills in a realistic manner.

COLLABORATIVE LEARNING EXPERIENCES IN HEALTH CARE

Types of collaborative learning experiences that can be designed in a simulation are variable and involve many different disciplines, practice settings, and health care scenarios. Examples of collaborative learning in health care settings are described below and summarized in Table 9-1.

Student to Student — In student to student collaboration, student learners or peers support one another's acquisition of knowledge and skills as a team. An example of this type of collaborative learning would be students practicing in pairs to learn how to take a blood pressure reading in preparation for a clinical demonstration. Wright (2003) provided a collaborative learning experience for nursing students in an environmental health class by pairing undergraduate students with graduate students from the School of Public Health. The 190 participants in the study concluded that the collaborative process was helpful. The group activities on environmental issues demonstrated how nursing students could function as members of a professional team, and knowledge of the environmental issues increased significantly ($p > .05$) after the collaborative activity. On the down side, however, this type of student to student collaboration can have a higher risk of not succeeding if the experience is driven by novices or is limited in faculty direction. For student to student collaboration to be successful, it also is important to match individuals' learning styles (Bonwell & Eison, 1991).

Faculty to Student — Faculty members are in a unique position to help motivate and shape students (Chickering & Gamson, 1987; Wilson, Gaff, Dienst, Wood, & Bavry, 1975). Through teacher-learner interactions such as simulated patient rounds by a group of health care students and the instructor, students can gain direction and validation from the expert. This support can encourage students to proceed in the learning process even when they encounter academic obstacles. In addition, students' values and belief systems are shaped through these types of relationships. In professional schools such as nursing, it is important for faculty and students to recognize that students are not only scholars or learners, but are future colleagues who will one day serve as mentors themselves (Childress, 2005). When objectives and goals are provided, the faculty to student pattern of interaction tends to have a greater success rate for active learning than student to student (Bonwell & Eison).

Academic Faculty to Clinicians/Clinical Faculty — Academic faculty in the simulated clinical setting can collaborate with clinicians in health care settings to establish an experience for students prior to their entering the clinical setting. Also, the virtual learning center can be used as an alternative learning environment for students who need additional experiences to help master process, integrate theory with practice in the actual clinical setting, manage patient care situations, and learn how to interact with patients and other health care professionals as a team. One example of this type of collaborative learning experience is incorporating simulations into clinical orientations. Another example is an academic faculty member working in the simulation setting with students who need additional help to master clinical skills while the clinical faculty member remains on the clinical unit with the other students. This model considers learners' needs and allows all learners to proceed at their own pace. It also provides a clinical group with the opportunity to continue their clinical experience in the simulation center. This collaborative model may be achieved by using simulated mannequins as patients and by gaining the assistance of clinicians.

Interdisciplinary — It is important when creating simulation scenarios to include professionals from a variety of health disciplines so students can identify appropriate responsibilities for each role and develop mutual respect for the contribution of each member of the health care team. Students from various disciplines (e.g., nursing and medical students, first-responders, others) can learn together how to manage resuscitation emergencies, terrorist events, rescue efforts, and routine health care situations. For example, Reese, Jeffries, and Engum (2006) conducted a study placing third-year medical students with senior nursing students to help them learn how to work together to provide care to a post-operative patient. The medical and nursing students worked together in a 20-minute simulation followed by a 20-minute debriefing. The patient in the scenario was a post-operative adult who developed acute chest pain, multi-focal PVCs, and eventual ventricular tachycardia. The learning outcomes measured in the study included teamwork, collaboration, and interdisciplinary communication. Likewise, Tucker, Wakefield, Boggis, Lawson, Roberts, and Gooch (2003) conducted a collaborative study assessing medical and nursing students working together to learn clinical skills in a uni-professional versus multi-professional group. Groups rotated through skill stations taught by multi-professional facilitators. The groups stayed together for a series of three sessions held at weekly intervals. The 113 third-year medical students and 43 diploma nursing students increased their confidence level with all skill sets encountered. Qualitative data provided evidence of the students' wish to learn in multi-professional groups versus uni-professional groups since feedback from the learning and shared knowledge and understanding were important dimensions of the project.

Table 9-1. Types of Collaborative Learning Experiences

Type	Description
Student to Student	Student learners or peers supporting one another's acquisition of knowledge and skills as a team.
Faculty to Student	Through teacher-learner interactions, students gain direction and validation from the expert.
Academic Faculty to Clinicians/Clinical Faculty	Academic faculty in the simulated clinical setting collaborate with clinicians in healthcare settings to establish pre-clinical and alternative clinical learning experience for students.
Interdisciplinary	Students from various disciplines learn together to manage various healthcare situations as a team, identify appropriate responsibilities for each role, and develop mutual respect for the contribution each makes to the team.

GOALS IN A COLLABORATIVE LEARNING ENVIRONMENT

In collaborative learning, the educator and students share goal setting. In the case of a simulation, the goals students desire to achieve from the simulation and the goals the educator hopes to meet both need to be considered.

Goals of the Educator

During a collaborative experience such as a simulation, the educator may desire that students understand interventions and problem solving pertaining to the care of a specific client and health disruption or a specific goal as described in the course syllabus. Whatever the goal, the educator generally has an outcome in mind. For example, the educator may have the goal that students are able to identify a basic arrhythmia and implement priority interventions to care for a patient experiencing this disorder. Goals with predictable answers are discussed in the debriefing sessions following the simulation. Open-ended goals have several avenues of inquiry that could produce a variety of unpredictable responses; open-ended goals usually motivate more lateral thinking and more widespread participation among group members. The achievement of this type of goal can also be accomplished in debriefing sessions or in the classroom.

Goals of the Learner

Learners should formulate their own goals based on the collaborative teaching-learning activity they plan to encounter. When students perceive that they are working to achieve their own goals as well as the educator's goals, they are more committed to the work of the simulation and the course (Hamilton). Students sharing their goals in a group help other group members with their goal achievement. Educators at times may need to assist students with their goal setting, since the goals will affect the nature of inquiry and activity within the simulated experience.

FACULTY ROLES IN COLLABORATIVE LEARNING SIMULATION EXPERIENCES

During a collaborative learning simulation experience, a faculty member may play a variety of roles in the teaching-learning environment. These roles are described below and are summarized in Table 9-2.

Table 9-2. Faculty Roles when Using Simulations in Nursing Education	
Role	**Description**
Patient or Other Member of the Care Team	Provides authenticity; consistency in the learning process
Facilitator	Guides but does not dictate the learning experience
Debriefer	Provides opportunities for student reflection on things that worked, did not work well, and how to improve; faculty provides expert knowledge during this process
Evaluator	Provides progress report on development of competence
Researcher	Seeks to answer questions regarding the use of simulation in nursing education

Patient or Other Member of the Care Team

In the role as standardized patient, the faculty member takes on the characteristics and physical condition with which a particular patient may present in order for the students to have an opportunity to practice and refine certain skills. For example, the faculty member could assume the role of an "ailing" geriatric client (including appearance and behaviors consistent with the script) from whom the student learner must obtain a health history. As a standardized patient, faculty may provide more authenticity to the situation because of their professional knowledge and experience (Lovell, Mavis, Turner, Ogle, & Griffith, 1998). Although assuming this role may be time-consuming, it may minimize the costs of recruiting and training lay individuals for this role. In addition, faculty members as standardized patients may be able to give a more consistent simulated learning experience as it is presented to each student. This, in turn, may improve students' acquisition of knowledge and skills.

The faculty member also might be assigned to the role of care team member. Johnson, Zerwic, and Theis (1999) assigned a faculty member to the role of a physician, where she/he would periodically receive phone calls from students who reported on a particular patient and conditions or problems. Again, the faculty member's expertise makes it possible to take on such a role quite effectively.

Facilitator

In the facilitator role, the faculty member serves as a guide rather than as a teacher; he/she is not directly dictating what learners need to do or determining a particular sequence the learners should use, but he/she provides the objectives for the collaborative learning experience. These objectives are used to guide or assist the students in working as a group when completing the simulation experience. When constructing a simulation scenario, it is important to provide students with a situation that requires them to utilize each other and to solve problems as a team. Providing opportunities for problem solving challenges students to examine personal perceptions of knowledge, to rely on each other to provide information, to establish a different view or framework based on exposure to diverse interpretations of available information, and to formulate a cooperative plan as to how to proceed as a group in order to solve the situation (Smith & MacGregor, 1992). One example of faculty taking on the role of facilitator is giving a simulation case study to a group of students and allowing them time to work through the problem of caring for the patient during a set time frame while being present in the room but not available to direct the process.

Debriefer

Once the simulation learning experience has been implemented, the learning experience is not complete until the students and faculty member have had an opportunity to reflect on the implementation process. During the reflection phase, students (and faculty) have the opportunity to identify how or whether decision making was appropriate as well as what areas need improvement. In the debriefer role, faculty members help students identify areas within the simulation where they did well, provide instruction for areas that have gaps, and provide students with support that will allow them to move forward in the learning process. Faculty in the role of debriefer are able to provide novices with expert knowledge and guidance. For example, students functioning in a mock code may be able to implement all the necessary steps to provide recovery for the patient. But they may not recognize that some of the steps should have been implemented in a different sequence to improve the effectiveness of their actions until after they have had an opportunity to reflect on the process and/or until the expert shares this information with them during the reflective thinking process. Nehring, Lashley, and Ellis (2002) discuss how faculty and students can solve problems and experiment with different solutions (e.g., "what if" scenarios) in a nonthreatening environment using simulations.

Evaluator

An important piece of the learning process is evaluation. It is important to assess and document competencies and skill sets. Students need feedback to determine whether or not they are on the right track. Validation is also needed to ensure safety of clients. Simulations can help teach theory and develop problem solving and clinical reasoning skills. Simulations also can help assess a student's performance progress when the simulation has been designed to measure competence (Salas & Burke, 2002; Satish & Streufert, 2002). It is important that faculty members in the role of evaluator help the novice acquire knowledge and appropriate behavioral skills.

Researcher

Faculty need to determine what works and what does not work in order to provide students with good learning experiences. An example of this is a pilot research study conducted to test the simulation design characteristics and educational practices embedded in the simulation framework (Jeffries, 2005). Findings from the study revealed collaboration and feedback/debriefing as important design features in constructing a simulation. This study supports many other claims identifying feedback/debriefing as an important component of simulations.

BENEFITS AND CHALLENGES OF COLLABORATIVE LEARNING IN SIMULATED EXPERIENCES

It is important to note that collaborative learning is an excellent way to foster student learning. Students and faculty have important roles to play in the collaborative learning process. There are several benefits and challenges that need to be addressed when considering incorporating collaborative learning experiences in simulation education.

Benefits of Collaborative Learning

Johnson and Johnson (1986) note that students working in groups achieve higher levels of thought, gain a deeper understanding of content, and are able to retain information longer than students who work individually. In addition, cooperative learning experiences provide opportunities for students to work together as a team to apply knowledge gained in the classroom setting as well as solve problems through discussion and reflection; the experiences help them develop critical thinking abilities (Gokhale; Rau & Heyl, 1990); assist them in coping with anxiety associated with the learning process (Gokhale); help them learn professional collaborative skills while working together; and improve confidence.

Collaborative learning experiences motivate students and promote "active learning." Active learning, a principle of best practices in education (Chickering & Gamson), encourages students to engage in the learning activities; focuses on developing students' abilities/skills during the process; provides opportunities that allow students to explore attitudes and values; increases student motivation to learn; provides opportunities for immediate feedback from the instructor; and fosters analytical thinking. Collaborative simulated learning provides a means of bridging the learning gap between generations. Incorporating collaborative learning experiences in simulation can provide students an opportunity to enhance their critical thinking through inclusion of problem-solving situations.

A simulated health care setting can provide an ideal active-learning environment that is safe, engaging, and realistic. Health care simulation scenarios (e.g., mock codes or resuscitation events) can be developed to allow students to work in teams. When functioning in a group, students collectively work together to solve problems and provide care during the simulated experience. During the group experience, students also have the opportunity to support each other during stressful situations. In this collaborative learning experience, students can reflect and analyze together what worked effectively and share ideas about areas where improvement may be necessary. Working in groups helps students learn from each other as well as develop and hone decision-making and critical-thinking skills.

Simulation allows students to assimilate isolated pieces of data and discern pertinent information from irrelevant information. Simulation activities also invite students to participate in groups when the learning experience is set up with this goal in mind. Sharing patient data helps them develop decision-making skills with decreased stress (Gokhale), since students are more comfortable sharing ideas in a group than in a faculty-student situation. When in groups, concepts can be clarified and problem solving implemented among peers and clinical instructors more easily than in a one-on-one situation with a clinical instructor. In addition, students have the opportunity to see how others solve problems.

As students work together to care for a patient in a collaborative simulated environment, they learn the responsibilities of other disciplines as well as how to function as a team member. Feedback from the educator/facilitator allows for more specific assessment of learning achievements and helps identify areas in which more knowledge and practice may be needed.

Challenges of Collaborative Learning

Challenges associated with collaborative simulated learning include having adequate and appropriate simulation equipment to promote active learning (Bonwell & Eison). Collaborative learning does not facilitate individual learning styles and "buy-in" for group learning needs to occur, especially from those who tend to be more individual learners. Another limitation is having adequate time to implement the simulation, including provision of instructions, the actual simulation, debriefing, and incorporating simulations into programs and courses. Other considerations that must be made include the following:

Individual Learning Styles — Gokhale examined the effectiveness of individual learning versus collaborative learning in enhancing drill-and-practice skills and critical-thinking skills. In a core collaborative learning environment, individual differences become part of the rich culture of the group rather than a detriment to any member of the group.

Leveling of Students — Matching leveling or learner capabilities is important to consider, as there may be concern about the additional time needed to bring less capable peers along. If the collaborative learning experience is structured so that all students are required to participate, then all can give help within the group as well as receive it. In this way, students of all abilities and different learning styles can work together effectively.

Group Selection — The level and type of student participating in the collaborative learning experience can improve participation and learning outcomes. There is a possibility however that some students may be more intellectually mature than others, and this may cause frustration if students such as these are expected to bear more group responsibilities than other students. According to Gokhale's research on relationships between collaborative learning and critical thinking, some students found they "wasted a lot of time explaining the material to other group members." According to Rau and Heyl, one needs to consider diversity, thinking styles, and expertise of individuals when determining group size. A small group (of three) may limit decision.

Group Size — Group size must promote active participation of team members and allow the group to maintain time on task and use time efficiently. Nehring and colleagues found that simulation groups larger than 8-10 students prevented students from adequately observing and interacting with the patient and simulation equipment.

Human Resources — Staff will be necessary to manage facilitation of processes as well as complete the reflective thinking process, especially since reflection is a key element of the simulation process.

Fair Grading — If the learning experience is to be graded, then a fair system for grading will need to be developed for group or collaborative performance.

Authenticity — Equipment and simulations need to be authentic in order to replicate practice situations learners will encounter in the clinical setting. Such authenticity enhances learning and facilitates transfer of learning from the simulation setting to the clinical setting.

Cost — Simulation design and development are initially time consuming and can be costly depending on the degree of realism. The cost of mannequins, props and other resources can be overwhelming. Various partnerships can help reduce these expenses. Costs may be borne by one institution but recovered by allowing other departments or institutions to use the resources for a fee. Some schools of nursing have already implemented this type of arrangement. Developing partnerships with agencies that have products necessary for student simulation learning is invaluable when designing and developing simulation programs.

SUMMARY

Students today are faced with huge amounts of information they are expected to learn (Linares, 1999). According to Skiba (2005), current college students, sometimes referred to as the "Net Generation" or the "Millennials," are more "hands-on," active learners, multitaskers and collaborators, who embrace technologies as an inherent part of how they communicate and learn. Millennials like to work in teams with peer-to-peer collaboration. All these individuals have different learning styles and require different educational modalities. Meeting those learning needs across the lifespan can be challenging for educators. Simulation in nursing education brings major considerations and challenges, but the benefits appear to outweigh the challenges. In an era when a shortage of nurses in both education and practice is the norm, the goal of increased collaboration may be difficult to achieve. However, if students are to graduate with beginning competency to function in community and interdisciplinary settings, they must participate in meaningful clinical experiences that promote the development of critical thinking skills and collaborative learning. More research needs to be conducted to evaluate the most effective way to incorporate simulation in collaborative learning experiences.

REFERENCES

Bonwell, C. C., & Eison, J. A. (1991). *Active learning: Creating excitement in the classroom.* (ASHE-ERIC Higher Education Report No. 1). Washington, DC: George Washington University.

Chickering, A.W., & Gamson, Z. F. (1987, March). Seven principles of good practice in undergraduate education. *AAHE Bulletin, 39*(7), 5-10.

Childress, R. M. (2005). An exploration of simulation in nursing education: A collaborative approach utilizing a mock code. *Virginia Nurses Today, 13*(4), 1-3.

Gokhale, A. A. (1995). Collaborative learning enhances critical thinking. *Journal of Technology Education, 7*(1), 1045-1064.

Hamilton, S. (1997). Collaborative learning. In *Teaching and learning in the arts, sciences, and professional schools* (pp. 3-9). Indianapolis, IN: IUPUI Center for Teaching and Learning.

Hamman, W. R. (2004, October). The complexity of team training: What we have learned from aviation and its applications to medicine. *Quality & Safety in Health Care, 13* (Suppl 1), 72-79.

Jeffries, P. R. (2005). A framework for designing, implementing, and evaluating simulations used as teaching strategies in nursing. *Nursing Education Perspectives, 26*(2), 96-103.

Johnson, R. T., & Johnson D. W. (1986). Action research: Cooperative learning in the science classroom. *Science and Children, 24*, 31-32.

Johnson, J. H., Zerwic, J. J., & Theis, S. L. (1999). Clinical simulation laboratory: An adjunct to clinical teaching. *Nurse Educator, 24*(5), 37-41.

Koerner, J. G. (2003). The virtues of the virtual world: Enhancing the technology/knowledge professional interface for life-long learning. *Nursing Administration Quarterly, 27*(1), 9-17.

Linares, A. Z. (1999). Learning styles of students and faculty in selected health care professions. *Journal of Nursing Education, 38*(9), 407–414.

Long, K. A. (2004). Preparing nurses for the 21st century: Reenvisioning nursing education and practice. *Journal of Professional Nursing, 20*(2), 82-88.

Lovell, K. L., Mavis, B. E., Turner, J. L, Ogle, K. S., & Griffith, M. (1998). Medical students as standardized patients in a second-year performance-based assessment experience. *Medical Education Online, 3*(6), 1-6.

Loyd, G. E., Lake, C. L., & Greenberg, R. B. (Eds.). (2004). *Practical health care simulations*. Philadelphia: Elsevier.

Maddox, P. J., Wakefield, M., & Bull, J. (2001). Patient safety and the need for professional and educational change. *Nursing Outlook, 49*(1), 8-13.

Nehring, W. M., Lashley, F. A., & Ellis, W. E. (2002). Critical incident nursing management using human patient simulators. *Nursing Education Perspectives, 23*(3), 128-132.

Rau, W., & Heyl, B. S. (1990). Humanizing the college classroom: Collaborative learning and social organizations among students. *Teaching Sociology, 18*, 141-155.

Reese, C., Jeffries, P. R., & Engum, S. (2006). Using simulations to develop educational experiences between nursing and medical students. Unpublished manuscript, Indiana University Schools of Nursing and Medicine, Indianapolis.

Salas, E., & Burke, C. S. (2002). Simulation for training is effective when... *Quality & Safety in Health Care, 11*, 119-120.

Satish, U., & Streufert, S. (2002). Value of a cognitive simulation in medicine: Towards optimizing decision making performance of healthcare personnel. *Quality & Safety in Health Care, 11*, 163–167.

Skiba, D. J. (2005). The Millennials: Have they arrived at your school of nursing? *Nursing Education Perspectives, 26*(6), 370-371.

Smith, B. L., & MacGregor, J. T. (1992). What is collaborative learning? In A. S. Goodsell, M. R. Maher, & V. Tinto (Eds.), *Collaborative learning: A sourcebook for higher education* (pp. 9-22). Syracuse, NY: National Center on Postsecondary Teaching, Learning, & Assessment, Syracuse University.

Tucker, K., Wakefield, A., Boggis, C., Lawson, M., Roberts, T., & Gooch, J. (2003). Learning together: Clinical skills for medical and nursing students. *Medical Education, 37*, 630-637.

Wilson, R. C., Gaff, J. G., Dienst, E. R., Wood, L., & Bavry, J. L. (1975). *College professors and their impact upon students.* New York: John Wiley & Sons.

Wright, D. J. (2003). Collaborative learning experiences for nursing students in environmental health. *Nursing Education Perspectives, 24*(4), 189-191.

Ziv, A., Wolpe, P. R., Small, S. D., & Glick, S. (2003). Simulation-based medical education: An ethical imperative. *Academic Medicine, 78*(8), 783-788.

CHAPTER 10
SUMMARY AND FUTURE CONSIDERATIONS

Mary Anne Rizzolo, EdD, RN, FAAN, Kristy Chambers, MSN, RN,
& Ruth Politi, MSN, RN

"In seeking knowledge, the first step is silence,

the second listening, the third remembering,

the fourth practicing,

and the fifth – teaching others."

Solomon Ibn Gabirol

Simulation in some form has probably been used as a teaching strategy in nursing education since the first nurse tried to teach the first nursing student how to do a task properly. As our understanding of teaching and learning progressed, so did the simulations that were used. Everyone who is reading this book can recall some experiences in the nursing school lab, perhaps positioning a mannequin, regulating an IV drip, or practicing blood pressure measurement on a fellow student. As audiovisual materials, then computers, were incorporated into the lab, slides, videos, and computer-assisted instruction programs were used to demonstrate skills prior to practice. These multifaceted experiences incorporating media, instruction by faculty, practice and return demonstrations, increased the amount of time that students spent in the lab.

Some innovative educators used the nursing lab in more creative ways, developing, for example, an experience in which the mannequin was an unconscious fresh post-op patient, and challenging students to do a quick assessment and discover such things as a name mismatch between the patient's armband and the chart, or "bleeding" from the abdominal incision, which could be seen only by the thorough student who turned the patient to his/her side. But, in general, most labs were used to practice skills.

Large learning resource centers began to appear in the late 1970s, when enterprising faculty in some schools secured funds from grants and other sources to build expansive centers containing equipment that was as good as or better than that which is found in most hospitals. Some purchased cameras to record student practice sessions, others had large audiovisual production capabilities, and still others used their funding to hire and train "standardized" patients, who described their health care problems and allowed students to practice physical examination and interviewing skills. But the advent of computerized mannequins and task trainers, and the decrease in the cost of that equipment, has brought us to a new era in the development and use of all kinds of simulations. This book, the first of its kind for nurse educators, was the work of an innovative, creative group of nurse educators who wished to share what they learned during the course of a three-year multisite project that tested simulation models and contributed to the refinement of the body of knowledge related to the use of simulation in nursing education.

Chapter 1. Using Simulation in Nursing Education provides some historical background on the use of simulations and the evolution of nursing as a practice-based discipline, one that is ideal for incorporating simulation as a teaching-learning activity. A definition of simulation is presented, and the advantages and challenges of developing simulations and incorporating them into the curriculum are explored, with examples provided from medicine and the military. A realistic overview of the challenges related to using simulations also is presented, including cost, space issues, faculty development needs, and time.

Chapter 2. Simulations: Education and Ethics offers strong arguments that simulation provides an excellent teaching and evaluation environment for students, and that nurse educators also should consider whether or not they have an ethical responsibility to provide simulated experiences to insure patient safety. Patient safety has been the subject of many studies, and simulation is discussed as a safe method for students to develop and maintain proficiency in a variety of skills, to practice interdisciplinary teamwork, to see immediately the positive outcomes of correct interventions, and to experience negative outcomes from incorrect decisions and errors in practice. The principles of justice, autonomy, beneficence, nonmaleficence, veracity, and compassion are discussed to argue for student experiences using simulations prior to clinical practice.

Chapter 3. Theoretical Framework for Simulation Design presents the advantages of using a framework that specifies relevant variables and their relationships to guide the design, implementation, and evaluation of simulations, and to conduct systematized research. The framework that was developed for the NLN/Laerdal Simulation Study (see Appendix A) is described, including the various learning theories that were considered in the early stages of the conceptualization of the framework. Each of the five components (teacher, student, educational practices, simulation design characteristics, and outcomes) is explained in detail, along with its relevance to simulations. Several areas for future research are proposed.

Chapter 4. Designing Simulations for Nursing Education. Faculty who have never developed a simulation often see it as a daunting task. The authors of this chapter use the familiar nursing process model to direct the development of a simulation, then provide an adaptable template to guide and assist in the simulation design process. The template contains essential areas such as learning objectives, prerequisite skills of students, and areas to describe the patient and his/her important diagnostic information and orders. It also includes practical check-off lists for assembling props and needed equipment, a section for predetermining student actions and cues as they move through a simulation, guided reflection questions, and ideas for varying the complexity of the simulation in the future. A list of the 2007 NCLEX-RN® Test Plan categories is included to assist faculty in tracking and matching student experiences with simulated patients to the test plan.

The completed template for the basic post-operative care scenario developed for the NLN/Laerdal Simulation Study (see Appendix A) also is provided. If faculty develop and share completed simulation templates, such as this one, the time for the creation of a simulation can be greatly reduced. While each simulation needs to reflect the specific learning objectives, content, and curricula at a given school, it is far easier to adapt an existing simulation than to create a new one, and templates can be regularly updated to reflect current evidence-based practice.

Chapter 5. Practical Suggestions for Implementing Simulations. Designing simulations and implementing them effectively requires passion, planning, creativity, and a willingness to change from traditional teacher-centered instruction to student-centered environments. This chapter describes the components required for effective execution of a well-prepared simulation: an appropriate venue or setting, a well thought out simulation design, a detailed script, clear directions and expectations, actors, props, rehearsals, technical support, feedback, evaluation, and expert time management. The authors then describe the phases of simulation implementation: (1) the scenario development process, (2) faculty/staff development and student orientation, (3) execution of the scenario, and (4) evaluation.

Chapter 6. Integrating Guided Reflection into Simulated Learning Experiences. This chapter begins with the philosophic underpinning of reflection, then proceeds to define reflection and the characteristics of reflective thinkers. The author discusses the work of experts in nursing who have written about the development of clinical judgment and reasoning, and the relationship of reflective thinking to this process. She explores both the positive and negative outcomes of reflective thinking and cites several frameworks and techniques that faculty can use to develop skill in conducting debriefing or reflective thinking sessions, particularly those that follow a simulated experience. Several tables are included that list guidelines for establishing a safe environment for reflection, the responsibilities of the facilitator, a tool for facilitating a reflection session, and research questions that need to be addressed.

Chapter 7. Evaluating Simulations. Evaluation of simulations can focus on the design of the simulation itself or measurement of the learner outcomes for which the simulation was created. Selected formative and summative evaluation strategies and how they can be incorporated into the evaluation of simulations are discussed in this chapter. First, the authors provide a description of the systematic process of conducting evaluation: identifying the purpose of the evaluation, determining a time frame, developing the plan, selecting appropriate instruments, collecting data, and interpreting data. Next, specific attention is devoted to evaluating the simulation activity itself. The Simulation Design Scale (SDS), a 20-item tool to evaluate the design and development phase, and the Educational Practices in Simulation Scale (EPSS), a 16-item tool that measures educational practices, provide examples of tools to evaluate the implementation phase of a simulation. Finally, a variety of studies that were conducted to measure learner outcomes are described, along with some of the tools that were used to measure knowledge and skills, learner satisfaction, critical thinking, and self-confidence.

Chapter 8. Setting Up a Simulation Laboratory. The Clinical Simulation Laboratory (CSL) is intended to replicate a "real world" clinical setting or situation as closely as possible. This chapter guides the reader on how to set up a CSL that will be efficient, flexible, cost-effective, and provide a rich teaching-learning environment. Whether building a new center or modifying existing space, this chapter is full of cost-saving ideas, advice, and helpful hints to assist with everything from assembling a design team and creating a floor plan, to the details of day-to-day operations, including scheduling and staffing suggestions, acquisition and maintenance of equipment and supplies, and inventory and restocking management.

A successful CSL has strong leadership, is staffed with appropriate personnel, and reflects strong institutional support, not only in the well-designed and constructed physical environment, but also in the support of faculty development regarding the design and implementation of simulations and their incorporation into the curriculum.

Chapter 9. Using Collaboration to Enhance the Effectiveness of Simulated Learning in Nursing Education. Today's complex health care environment requires collaboration and communication among the health care team to ensure quality patient care. Simulation in health care education is emerging and evolving as an effective way to facilitate this collaboration and communication process. Examples of the various types of collaborative learning experiences are described, including student to student, faculty to student, academic faculty to clinicians, and interdisciplinary exercises. The variety of roles that faculty can play when a simulation is designed to promote collaboration are discussed. Faculty will encounter many challenges when developing and coordinating a meaningful collaborative learning experience, but potential benefits for learners and the patients they will care for make the effort worthwhile.

CONCLUDING THOUGHTS

The chapters in this book have presented many advantages for using simulations in the education of tomorrow's nurses. Some of the most compelling reasons include

- Providing a safe, risk-free environment where students can practice without the fear of harming a client.
- Supplying every student with an opportunity to rehearse low frequency, high-risk clinical experiences that they would otherwise never experience.

- Ensuring that every student has the knowledge and skills to care for patients with commonly occurring health care problems.

- Practicing collaboration with other health care providers, leadership, and delegation skills.

- Allowing a student to safely experience and work through feelings around sensitive, uncomfortable and/or controversial situations they may encounter in practice (e.g., abortion, addicted or abused clients, and clients/families who are dealing with end-of-life issues).

When we immerse students in a scenario where they must use all their skills to assess a patient, then formulate and implement a plan of care, they become aware of the gaps in their knowledge — a sobering experience and a powerful motivator for learning.

Obviously more research is needed on simulations — to answer relatively simple questions, such as how much time is appropriate for a specific simulation or for a specific level of student — as well as to explore more complex questions, such as whether the use of simulations throughout the curriculum leads to better critical thinking and clinical judgment skills in graduates. Researchers also might explore whether a simulated experience prior to clinical practice lead to less anxiety and more learning during clinical experiences with patients, or how much clinical experience time can be replaced with simulated experiences in a specific course. The rich qualitative data that surfaces when students tell faculty about their experiences with simulation continues to generate more complex research questions.

Any type of research on educational strategies and practice is difficult. There are many challenges, and it is impossible to control some variables such as past experiences of students. Our evaluation instruments are limited. We have no good tools, for example, to measure the application of knowledge to care of a client, which is often the real purpose of a simulated experience. We must advance the science of nursing education to confront these challenges and inform our teaching practice.

Today's students have grown up with technology. They expect and deserve student-centered teaching and learning that incorporates the latest technological advancements to help them learn efficiently, effectively, and safely so they can provide quality care to patients. And technology is advancing at an increasingly rapid pace. Consider how quickly we have progressed from the simple computer-assisted instruction programs of the 1980s to virtual hospitals and complex patient situations with multiple paths and branches. The mannequins of today will be wireless tomorrow, they will walk as well as talk, and they will simulate sophisticated symptoms like changes in skin texture and sensation. Soon we will be able to immerse our students in a virtual health care environment, complete with entire units filled with patients and other health care personnel, complete with all of the sights, sounds and smells unique to that environment. Will faculty be prepared to harness and shape the learning environments of tomorrow and create meaningful learning, evidence-based experiences for their students? We hope this book can provide a beginning pathway to help faculty work toward that goal.

APPENDIX A
FINAL REPORT OF THE NLN/LAERDAL SIMULATION STUDY

Project Title

Designing and Implementing Models
for the Innovative Use of Simulation
to Teach Nursing Care of Ill Adults and Children:
A National, Multi-Site, Multi-Method Study

Project Sponsors

National League for Nursing and Laerdal Medical

Report Prepared by:

Pamela R. Jeffries, DNS, RN, FAAN, Project Director
Associate Professor and Associate Dean for Undergraduate Programs
Indiana University School of Nursing

Mary Anne Rizzolo, EdD, RN, FAAN
Senior Director for Professional Development
National League for Nursing

Project Period

June 1, 2003 to May 31, 2006

PURPOSES OF THE PROJECT

The purposes of this national, multi-site, multi-method project were fourfold:

1) To develop and test models that nursing faculty can implement when using simulation to promote student learning,

2) To develop a cadre of nursing faculty who can use simulation in innovative ways to enhance student learning,

3) To contribute to the refinement of the body of knowledge related to the use of simulation in nursing education, and

4) To demonstrate the value of collaboration between the corporate and not-for-profit worlds.

GOALS OF THE RESEARCH

The research goals were to explore how to design simulations, implement simulations as a teaching strategy, and evaluate selected learning outcomes using simulations. Specifically, the study was designed to:

1) Develop a teaching-learning framework incorporating simulations that nurse educators can use to help guide the development, implementation, and evaluation of the use of simulations in nursing education.

2) Describe and test a design that is theoretically based and can be used to develop nursing simulations that promote good learning outcomes.

3) Explore relationships among the theoretical concepts of the simulation framework to assess the existence and importance of these concepts.

4) Test and analyze selected outcomes when implementing a nursing simulation based on the proposed theoretical concepts using an experimental design.

PROJECT PHASES

Phase I: June 2003 to December 2003

The aim of this phase was to organize the eight Project Coordinators and one Project Director to discuss the project and set specific directions for the study. Specifically, Phase I was designed to clarify the purpose of the study; discuss the nature of participating in a national, multi-site study; conduct a review of the simulation literature; apply for IRB approval at each institution to conduct the research study there; develop a research design for each institution's specific simulation study using the research design, parameters, and essential elements defined by the project group; and discuss the specific and overall project goals and research with the Project Director during individual site visits.

Activities during the first six months of the project began with the selection of the Project Director and eight project sites, followed by a kickoff meeting to clarify goals and responsibilities, explore the theoretical framework for the research design, and explain the process for implementing the research over the three years of the project. After completing a comprehensive literature review to identify gaps in the simulation literature, a simulation framework was developed and the 4-phase research design was formulated. Since existing measurement tools were determined to be inadequate for the purposes of this study, new research instruments were developed during Phase I.

Phase II: January 2004 to June 2004

Phase II was designed to allow each Project Coordinator and her faculty colleagues to have first-hand experience designing a simulation within the parameters of the framework, implementing that simulation, and evaluating its effectiveness. As a result of these efforts, study participants were able to assess what worked well, define ideal timeframes for various components of the learning experience, obtain reliability and validity data on the instruments constructed to measure the concepts in the simulation teaching-learning framework, and develop a medical-surgical simulation that would be implemented across all eight sites during Phases III and IV.

Each Project Coordinator implemented a small simulation study at her school, with six sites using SimMan®, one site using an IV simulator, and one site using a low-fidelity mannequin. All sites used the Educational Practices in Simulation Scale (EPSS) and the Simulation Design Scale (SDS) to gather data about the experience.

The Project Director reviewed the curriculum at all eight sites and determined that every school taught basic care of the post-operative adult patient in the first clinical course. This content was selected, therefore, for the scenario that was designed for implementation across all sites during Phase III of the study.

Phase III: July 2004 to July 2005

Phase III consisted of two parts. Part 1 focused on obtaining baseline data about students' understanding of post-operative content before the teaching simulation was integrated. Part 2 focused on learning outcomes at the project sites when three different types of simulations were incorporated.

During Phase III, Part 1 (July to December 2004), baseline data about current practices and learning outcomes in medical-surgical courses where postoperative content is taught were obtained prior to implementing the study's simulation. The study design was then pilot tested at one site. This activity helped the group refine the simulation scenario, refine the research design, and obtain additional reliability and validity data on the instruments.

Three hundred ninety five students (female=350; male=45) completed a 12-item multiple choice pretest, and viewed a 38-minute videotaped lecture presented by an experienced master teacher who included a simulation of care of a postoperative adult patient. Following the lecture, students completed a 12-item parallel form posttest on postoperative care, the EPSS, the SDS, an instrument that measured their satisfaction with the instructional method, a self-confidence scale that measured their perceptions of their confidence in caring for a postoperative client, and a self-perceived judgment performance measure that provided information about students' perceptions of their clinical performance in the simulation.

In Phase III, Part 2 (January to July 2005), project sites implemented the standardized simulation focusing on care of a post-operative adult patient, using randomized control and experimental groups. Each then assessed the simulation design and process, using the SDS and EPSS; each evaluated selected learning outcomes for students experiencing three different types of simulations; and each assessed student satisfaction with the use of simulation as a teaching/learning strategy. Specific research questions addressed during Phase III, Part 2 of the study were as follows:

1) Will students who participate in the simulation as part of the teaching/learning experience related to care of an adult post-operative patient have better learning outcomes (knowledge, self-confidence, satisfaction, judgment performance) based on the type of simulation experienced (paper/pencil case study simulation, static mannequin, or high-fidelity patient simulator)?

2) Will there be differences regarding learning outcomes (knowledge, self-confidence, judgment performance, and learner satisfaction) based on the role assigned to a student in the simulation?

Four hundred three students who were enrolled in their first medical-surgical nursing course participated in this phase. These students were largely female (87%) and Caucasian (77%, with 8% self reporting as African American and 6% self reporting as Asian), and their average age was 29. Sixty-two percent were enrolled in baccalaureate programs, and 38% were students in associate degree programs. All participants completed the 12-item pretest on postoperative care and viewed a 38-minute videotape that included (a) a lecture by an experienced master teacher on the care of the postoperative adult patient and (b) a simulation demonstrating care of such a patient. Students were then randomly assigned to one of three types of simulation groups, each of which focused on care of a post-operative adult patient.

- One group was given a paper/pencil case study simulation. Students worked in groups of four to answer the questions and solve the problems presented.

- A second group participated in a hands-on simulated experience using a static mannequin.

- The third group also had a hands-on experience, but they used a high-fidelity patient simulator.

All three groups were provided the same simulation, worked in groups of four, and each group's simulation was conducted for 20 minutes. All students then participated in a 20-minute reflective thinking session immediately following the simulation that was either audio taped or videotaped. This guided reflection session was facilitated by the instructor who had observed the simulation, using specific scripted questions. Students then completed the EPSS and SDS as well as a test of their knowledge, the self-confidence scale, the judgment performance scale regarding their participation in the simulation, and a satisfaction survey.

In all instances, data collection took no longer than 30 minutes. Finally, in order to ensure that no students were disadvantaged because of the group to which they were assigned, all had an opportunity, prior to completion of the unit/module that included post-operative care of the adult surgical patient, to participate in the two types of simulations they had missed; none, however, took advantage of this opportunity.

Phase IV: August 2005 to June 2006

After analyzing data obtained in Phase III, the project team realized that since students only participated in one of the three types of simulations, their responses on data collection instruments were limited to the learning context they experienced (i.e., paper/pencil case study simulation, static mannequin, or high-fidelity patient simulator). Phase IV was designed, therefore, to expose all participating students to two different types of simulations, namely paper/pencil case study simulation and high-fidelity patient simulator, so they could compare the experiences. The same post-operative adult patient simulation that had been designed for Phase III of the study was used in Phase IV, and an alternate paper/pencil case study simulation was designed to parallel the high-fidelity patient simulator experience as much as possible and reflect similar content and levels of decision making. All other procedures and evaluation measures were the same as in Phase III, Part 2.

Two of the eight study sites participated in Phase IV. Half of the participating students (N=55; 86% female) worked with the paper/pencil case study simulation first and then worked with the high-fidelity patient simulator. The other half of the students (N=55; 86% female) participated in the simulation using the high-fidelity patient simulator first and then worked with the paper/pencil case study simulation. The following research questions guided this phase of the study:

1) Is there a difference in learner satisfaction when two different types of simulations are used by learners rather than when each student uses only one type?

2) Is there a difference in students' perceived presence and importance of educational practices when two different types of simulations are used by learners rather than when each student uses only one type?

3) Is there a difference in students' perceived presence and importance of simulation design factors when two different types of simulations are used by learners rather than when each student uses only one type?

4) Is there a difference in student self confidence when two different types of simulations are used by learners rather than when each student uses only one type?

5) Is there a difference in students' judgment of their performance when two different types of simulations are used by learners rather than when each student uses only one type?

The outcome measure of knowledge, using a multiple choice pre and posttest was eliminated in this phase since non-significant findings were obtained in the previous study using this measure.

INSTRUMENTS

The instruments used in the project included several questionnaires, some of which were specifically designed for the study and some of which were already in existence. Each instrument is described, and content validity and reliability determined during Phase III of the study are provided for each.

The *Simulation Design Scale (SDS)*, a 20-item instrument using a five-point scale, was designed to evaluate the five design features of the instructor-developed simulations used in this study. The five design features include objectives/information, support, problem solving, feedback, and fidelity. The instrument has two parts: one asks about the presence of specific features in the simulation, and the other asks about the importance of those features to the learner. Content validity for the SDS was established by ten content experts in simulation development and testing. The instrument's reliability was tested using Cronbach's alpha, which was found to be 0.92 for presence of features, and 0.96 for the importance of features.

The *Educational Practices in Simulation Scale (EPSS)*, a 16-item instrument using a five-point scale, was designed to measure whether four educational practices (active learning, collaboration, diverse ways of learning, and high expectations) are present in the instructor-developed simulation, and the importance of each practice to the learner. The educational practices were derived from the work of Chickering and Gamson (1987). Reliability was tested using Cronbach's alpha and was found to be 0.86 for the presence of specific practices and 0.91 for the importance of specific practices.

The Student Satisfaction with Learning Scale is a 5-item instrument designed to measure student satisfaction with five different items related to the simulation activity. Content validity of the instrument was established by nine clinical experts validating the content and relevance of each item for the concept of satisfaction. Reliability was tested using Cronbach's alpha and found to be 0.94.

The Self-Confidence in Learning Using Simulations Scale is an 8-item instrument measuring how confident students felt about the skills they practiced and their knowledge about caring for the type of patient presented in the simulation. Content validity was established by nine clinical experts in nursing, and reliability, tested using Cronbach's alpha, was found to be 0.87.

Cognitive Gain or Knowledge was measured by comparing scores on multiple choice tests related to caring for a post-operative adult patient. Two parallel forms of the test were designed by a test development expert to mimic NCLEX-RN® type questions. One form of the test was given prior to students' participation in any simulation, and the other form was given after completion of the simulation. Content validity of these tests was established by three experienced faculty.

The Self-Perceived Judgment Performance Scale is a 20-item-scale modified from the Judgment Performance Scale (Facione & Facione, 1998) used to measure higher order thinking in individuals during a performance. This scale was based on students' self-perception of their performance in the simulation as scored on a 5-point Likert Scale. The higher the score, the better the student perceived her/himself as performing appropriately and effectively within the simulation. Content validity of the modified scale was determined by nine clinical experts, and Cronbach's alpha established a 0.90 reliability for the scale.

Findings

Data from Phase II revealed that the prominent educational practice embedded in the simulations was that of collaboration. The most important simulation design feature was found to be feedback/debriefing.

Data from Phase III, Part I indicated that knowledge was gained by students in the traditional learning environment. Using a paired t-test, there was a significant difference ($p < .0001$) between the pre and posttest scores, indicating learning took place. The educational practices found to be embedded in the traditional instruction were active learning, collaboration, diverse ways of learning, and high expectations. High expectations was the educational practice that received the highest rating by students indicating they perceived this educational practice to be most present in the classroom experience. Overall, students were satisfied with the traditional approach to learning about caring for a postoperative adult patient, and they indicated that this experience helped them gain confidence in their ability to care for a postoperative patient.

When comparing data obtained from the 403 students during Phase III, Part 2, responses on the Simulation Design Scale (SDS) revealed the following:

- The group that used the high-fidelity patient simulator reported a greater sense of reality than did students in the other two groups, and the paper/pencil case study simulation group reported the least sense of reality

- The group that used the paper/pencil case study simulation was less likely than the other two groups to report they received feedback, but there was no significant difference on this aspect of the simulation design in the other two groups indicating those two types of simulations (static mannequin and high-fidelity patient simulator) provide similar feedback from the instructor to students

- The groups that used the static mannequin simulation or high-fidelity patient simulator reported more opportunities to problem-solve and make decisions in the simulation than did the paper/pencil case study simulation group

- Feedback was viewed as less important to the paper/pencil case study simulation group than it was to the other two groups

When comparing data obtained from the 403 students participating in Phase III, Part 2 of the study, responses on the Educational Practices in Simulation Scale (EPSS) revealed the following:

- The group that used the high-fidelity patient simulator reported a greater sense of being involved in diverse ways of learning than did students in the other two groups, and they valued this educational practice more than did students in those other groups

- The group that used the paper/pencil case study simulation agreed, more so than the other two groups, that collaboration was part of their simulation

- The group that used the paper/pencil case study simulation perceived higher expectations to perform well in the learning situation than did the group that used the static mannequin simulation

- Students who participated in either simulator group (static mannequin or high-fidelity patient simulator) perceived a greater presence of active learning and rated active learning as being more important in their learning experience than did the students who worked with the paper/pencil case study simulation

When comparing data obtained from the 403 students during Phase III, Part 2, responses on the 2-item, multiple choice, NCLEX-RN® type exam revealed that there were no significant differences in knowledge gains among the three groups as measured by pre and post testing, using Kruskal-Walis non-parametric tests (non-parametric version of the ANOVA) between each pair of groups. This is not a surprising finding, however, since students were not expected to acquire new knowledge during this experience. The simulations were designed to give them an opportunity to apply their knowledge, as learning with simulations should be directed toward synthesis and application of knowledge, rather than toward new knowledge development.

When comparing data obtained from the 403 students during Phase III, Part 2 of the study, responses on the Satisfaction Scale revealed that the group using the high-fidelity patient simulator had a significantly higher level of satisfaction with their learning experience than did students in the two other groups.

When comparing data obtained from the 403 students during Phase III, Part 2 of the study, responses on the Self-Confidence Scale revealed that students in the high-fidelity patient simulator and static mannequin simulation groups reported significantly greater confidence about their ability to care for a postoperative adult patient than did students in the paper/pencil case study simulation group.

When comparing data obtained from the 403 students during Phase III, Part 2 of the study, responses on the Self-Perceived Judgment Performance Scale revealed no significant difference among the three groups regarding their performance. It appears that students self-evaluate based on the context of the learning situation. If they achieved the stated objectives, and felt good about their participation, then they rated themselves as performing well.

Students who worked with the high-fidelity patient simulator or the static mannequin were randomly assigned to one of four roles: Nurse 1, Nurse 2, significant other, or observer. Students who participated in the paper/pencil case study simulation were not given roles. Data obtained during Phase III, Part 2 of the study revealed the following about the roles played:

- Regardless of the role they assumed during the simulation, there were no significant differences in knowledge gain among students

- Regardless of the role they assumed during the simulation, there were no significant differences in satisfaction or self-confidence regarding caring for a postoperative adult patient among students

- Students who assumed the Nurse 1 role rated themselves significantly higher on their judgment when caring for a postoperative adult patient when compared to those who assumed the Nurse 2 role

- Students who assumed the significant other role rated themselves significantly higher on their judgment when caring for a postoperative adult patient when compared to those who assumed the Nurse 2 role

- Students who assumed the observer role rated themselves significantly lower on their judgment when caring for a postoperative adult patient when compared to those who assumed the Nurse 2 role

- There were no significant differences on judgment when caring for a postoperative adult patient between those who assumed the role of Nurse 1 and those who assumed the role of significant other

When comparing data obtained from the 110 students (86% female; mean age of 26) who participated in Phase IV, responses on the Educational Practices in Simulation Scale (EPSS) and the Simulation Design Scale (SDS) revealed the following:

- Students in the high-fidelity patient simulator group reported active learning to be present and important significantly more often than did students in the paper/pencil case study simulation group

- Diverse ways of learning was rated higher by students in the high-fidelity patient simulator group than by those in the paper/pencil case study simulation group

- The paper/pencil case study simulation group rated collaboration and higher expectations significantly higher than did the high-fidelity patient simulator group

- The high-fidelity patient simulator group rated the importance of fidelity, presence of feedback, support, and objectives significantly higher than did the paper/pencil case study simulation group

- Overall, students in the high-fidelity patient simulator group were significantly more satisfied with their learning activity than were students in the paper/pencil case study simulation group

- The high-fidelity patient simulator group rated themselves significantly more confident and satisfied with the instruction than did the paper/pencil case study simulation group

- The paper/pencil case study simulation group judged their performance significantly higher than did the high-fidelity patient simulator group

CONCLUSIONS

Based on findings that the paper/pencil case study simulation group did not perceive as many problem-solving features or opportunities to problem-solve in their learning experience as the other two groups did, one can conclude that the more active the learning experience, the more important feedback is to the learner. Feedback facilitates the decision-making/problem-solving process; thus, paper/pencil case study simulations may be less effective than other types of simulations in helping students develop these skills that are critical for clinical practice. Perhaps the difference can be attributed to the fact that a case study provides information about a patient while active involvement in a simulation requires students to discover and make sense of that information for themselves.

Based on findings that students in both simulator groups (i.e., static mannequin and high-fidelity) placed higher value on diverse ways of learning and active learning than did students in the paper/pencil case study simulation, one can conclude that students' judgments about the importance of various educational practices are influenced by the learning context in which they are placed. If learners are not exposed to diverse and active educational practices, they do not know what they have missed and may not value those practices.

Based on the findings that the group using the high-fidelity patient simulator had a significantly higher level of satisfaction with their learning experience than did students in the two other groups, one can conclude that high-fidelity patient simulator experiences incorporate more of the principles of best practice in education as described by Chickering and Gamson (1987).

Based on the findings that there were no significant difference among the three groups regarding their perceived performance, one can conclude that students evaluate themselves based on the context of the learning situation, not on the objectives to be attained. In other words, if they achieved the stated objectives and felt good about their participation, then they rated themselves as performing well.

Based on findings related to knowledge gain, confidence, satisfaction, and various roles assumed in a simulation (i.e., Nurse 1, Nurse 2, significant other, or observer), one can conclude that role assignment does not affect overall student learning outcomes. It is important to note that since those assigned to the observer role did not rate collaboration highly on the EPSS, faculty may need to structure the learning experience to provide some mechanism for students in this role to engage in collaborative work.

Based on findings related to student satisfaction with their learning experience, one can conclude that high-fidelity patient simulator experiences incorporate more of the principles of best practice in education as described by Chickering and Gamson (1987).

Based on findings related to self-confidence, one can conclude that learning through paper/pencil case study simulation is not as effective in promoting confidence in students since that experience lacks realistic, timely opportunities for students to "test" themselves in providing care to patients.

Based on the findings related to performance, one can conclude that paper/pencil case study simulations may help students perceive a greater level of performance because they are more experienced with the case study method of learning.

Students who participated in paper/pencil case study simulations believed that their instructors had high expectations of them and their experience promoted collaborative learning. However, this approach provided less fidelity, fewer opportunities for problem solving, and fewer opportunities for providing feedback to students.

Overall, students who worked with the high-fidelity patient simulator were more satisfied with the instructional method and reported greater confidence in their ability to care for a postoperative adult patient. More than other students, this group believed that their experience provided for more fidelity and feedback, and they rated those design features as the most important ones. With regard to educational practices incorporated into a simulation experience, students whose experience incorporated the high-fidelity patient simulator perceived significantly more active learning and diverse ways of learning than did other students, and they rated active learning as the most important educational practice. Furthermore, these students seemed to learn and be satisfied even when they played roles other than that of "nurse" in a simulation.

Summary

The findings of this national, multi-site, multi-method study on *Designing and Implementing Models for the Innovative Use of Simulation to Teach Nursing Care of Ill Adults and Children* support those reported in the literature on simulations, even though that literature base is somewhat limited. It is clear that the educational practices and simulation design characteristics in the simulation framework are relevant and important to incorporate into simulations in order to provide a quality learning experience for students. In addition, the simulation framework has been found to be valuable as a guide for conducting systematic, organized research on simulations.

While more research is needed, it appears that immersion in a simulation provides the opportunity to apply and synthesize knowledge in a realistic but non-threatening environment. Active involvement and the opportunity to apply observational, assessment, and problem-solving skills, followed by a reflective thinking experience, leads to increased self-confidence in students. In addition, when students are more active and immersed in a learning situation, the feedback they receive regarding what they did correctly and incorrectly can greatly facilitate their learning. It is expected that the expanded use of simulation in nursing education will facilitate increased learning and skill transfer when students care for patients in today's complex, health care environment.

REFERENCE

Chickering, A. W., & Gamson, Z. F. (1987, March). Seven principles of good practice in undergraduate education. <u>AAHE Bulletin,</u> <u>39</u>(7), 5-10.

Facione, N.C., & Facione, P.A. (1998). <u>Professional Judgment Rating Form</u>. Millbrae, CA: The California Press.

APPENDIX B
AUTHOR PROFILES